SACRED HEALING

SACRED HEALING

The Curing Power
of Energy and
Spirituality

C. NORMAN SHEALY
M.D., PH.D.

ELEMENT
Boston, Massachusetts • Shaftsbury, Dorset
Melbourne, Australia

© Element Books, Inc. 1999
Text © Norman Shealy, M.D., Ph.D. 1999

First published in the USA in 1999 by
Element Books, Inc.
160 North Washington Street
Boston, Massachusetts 02114

Published in Great Britain in 1999 by
Element Books Limited
Shaftesbury, Dorset SP7 8BP

Published in Australia in 1999 by
Element Books Limited for
Penguin Books Australia Limited
487 Maroondah Highway, Ringwood, Victoria 3134

The selection on pages 19–21 originally published by Dr. Marcus Bach,
Fellowship for Spiritual Understanding.
Reproduced by permission of Mrs. Marcus Bach.

Library of Congress Cataloging-in-Publication data

Shealy, C. Norman, 1932–
     Sacred healing : the curing power of energy and spirituality / C.
Norman Shealy.
          p. cm.
     Includes bibliographical references.
     ISBN 1-86204-377-9 (alk. paper)
     1. Alternative medicine. 2. Therapeutics, Suggestive. 3. Mind and body. 4.
Health—Religious aspects. 5. Spirituality—Health aspects. I. Title.
R733.S533 1999
615.8'52—dc21   99-17673
                                                          CIP

British Library Cataloguing in Publication data avalable

Book design by Jill Winitzer
Printed and bound in the United States by Courier

ISBN 1-86204-377-9

Contents

Foreword

Healing, by definition, is a sacred art. Practically all of the ancient texts describe the art of healing as a divine process in which healing the body first requires healing the spirit. When the potential of technical and chemical medicine accelerated during the second half of this century, the "spirit" of healing was made ill. That is, the consciousness that healing is a sacred art was eclipsed by a more scientific modality. Though not a deliberate intention on the part of the scientific community, respect for the healing power of prayer, faith and love diminished dramatically as chemical medicine produced more and more physical results.

The one of these three internal qualities that retained a position of respect within the allopathic medical community was faith. Even then, the energy of faith had to be directed toward supporting the potential healing technologies of the allopathic community. The healing power of faith was reduced to a personal matter that carried little or no authority in the external world. It seemed that as the scientific and medical community accelerated in its growth and development, faith became a property of a more religious arena.

The entry of the scientific mind into the medical world has been and remains essential. The research done in these past five decades has been a masterful contribution to the knowledge we need to have about the chemistry and physiology of our own bodies. But somewhere along the line, the precious role of the Sacred has been reduced to the status of superstition and non-provable thought, dropped completely from the list of significant factors that contribute to health or the disintegration of health.

The information in this book, *Sacred Healing*, looks at the interior of the human soul and honors its position of power within the human body. C. Norman Shealy, M.D., Ph.D., leads the reader into the history of sacred healing, beginning with the ancient Romans and Greeks. This journey examines the role of religion and religious rituals that revolve around healing as well as the sacred sites that emerged during that time. Shealy also introduces the reader to contemporary sacred healing and the research that has been done to study the effects of sacred techniques such as prayer and the laying on of hands.

Typical of Shealy's ability to draw together numerous angles into one unified pattern, he presents an insightful view of the challenges that the contemporary healer faces within his culture. He discusses his own search for authentic healers that began in 1972 and took him to various cultures and spiritual traditions. The knowledge that he gained along the way is an encyclopedia unto itself. This incredible book is a product of his own personal journey as well as the sojourns of gifted healers who report on their successes and failures.

I have personally known Norm since 1984. While I recognize that he is a brilliant physician, I think of him first as the quintessential research scientist whose primary interest in this life is to discover more about the relationship of the energy—or sacred texture of the human being—to the physical body. This is his life's passion, and this passion is evident in every page of this book. Norm has thoroughly investigated, and continues to investigate, alternative sacred healing techniques, such as electromagnetic healing and psychic surgery. In this book, he shares his years of personally investigating some of the most prominent energy healers of our time, describing their techniques and their successes.

Norm knew (and knows) many of these healers, and he writes about them with clarity and discernment.

For all of us who are interested in understanding the nature of healing, this book is a necessary part of our library. It is becoming increasingly evident that the themes of this next millennium are healing and the emergence of the sacred into the entire weave of life, and C. Norman Shealy has performed a valuable service by writing *Sacred Healing*.

Caroline M. Myss, Ph.D.

Introduction:
What Is Sacred
Healing?

What is sacred healing? You have heard of spiritual healing, but sacred? What's the difference?

Spiritual is "of, relating to, or concerned with the soul or spirit" according to *Webster's New Lexicon Dictionary*. Spirit is "The intelligent or immaterial part of a human as distinguished from the body"—"The animating or vital principle" of life.

Sacred means "holy," "consecrated," or related to "worship of God." The spirit is part of that which is created by God, but sacred implies a reverence for God itself. And if you are Theist, one who believes in God, then sacred implies a reverence for all things created by God. Thus, sacred includes a reverence for life itself, for the principles of life and for all that sustains life. In this sense, all healing is sacred, and all therapies intended for healing are sacred. Indeed, every aspect of the universe is sacred!

Sacred includes all aspects of mysticism and religion. But something is sacred only when it is noetic, or "ineffable" to the individual, beyond explanation. William James, in *The Varieties of Religious Experience*, emphasized the importance of mystical states of consciousness. All of them are part of consciousness. Mysticism, thus, encompasses truth, deception, pleasure and pain. Mysticism is the experience of the sacred.

What William James called "the mind-cure movement," which began with Mary Baker Eddy and Christian Science, encompasses only one aspect of healing. One of my most profound experiences occurred when I was a senior resident of neurosurgery at the Massachusetts General Hospital. One evening, a man brought his comatose sister into the hospital emergency room. An emergency X-ray of the arteries to the brain demonstrated a moderate tumor in the right frontal lobe, and I removed that tumor, which turned out to be a metastatic squamous cell carcinoma. The woman recovered consciousness overnight. The primary cancer was found to be an exquisitely small tumor in the urethra, and it was apparently cured with radiation.

During the days after her recovery, however, she was

extremely agitated and weepy, and one day I said, "If you do not improve your attitude, you will never get well." She replied, "Oh, Dr. Shealy, are you a Christian Scientist, too?" Her agitation had to do with the fact that she had failed to cure herself and had succumbed to medical treatment, including surgery. I explained to her that I considered all aspects of healing, including medical and surgical therapy, to be God-given.

Spiritual healing has traditionally been considered a miraculous type of healing that occurs usually through the laying on of hands, originally by kings or priests, but in modern times by a number of religious and spiritually oriented practitioners. Kathryn Kuhlman, Oral Roberts and the most studied of all, Ambrose and Olga Worrall, are but a few of these modern "healers." Some, like Sally Hammond, have taken it further and considered that "we are all healers." In many respects, I would agree with her.

In a sense, religion is often practiced as a petition to God. Metaphysically oriented individuals believe in the power of positive thinking or affirmation, and a truly mystical God. God-oriented individuals believe in receiving the power of God.

Mystics believe in guidance from God, either by intuitive insights, or messages from angels, or the soul. They also accept the sacred nature of all aspects of life and an evolution of consciousness toward that which is more in harmony with the will of God. Belief, attitude, positive thinking, prayer, are all magnetic attractions, a result of an attitude of the sacred.

Edgar Cayce perhaps expressed the universal sacred nature of healing best when he said "There is no difference, for the good in each treatment comes from the same source. They are not contradictory, as some people believe."[1] He goes on to say, "In every realm, then, of mind, body and soul, there is an entombment to that oneness." Or, "All healing comes from the divine." And, finally, "Perhaps, in reality, the doctor, psychologist, and priest are the workers at the same laboratory table, the molders of the same ductile clay, three tenders of the same divine fire."[2]

When the body was separated from the soul by Descartes, modern scientific medicine began. Unfortunately, during the two-century period since then, not only the spiritual but the sacred have been ignored to a large extent by the medical profession. Thus, most people have forgotten the connectedness of all healing to the God-force itself.

Essentially, everything in the universe as we understand it is energy, manifesting in light and/or sound. We are unable to measure the subtle energy of a soul or the spirit of God itself.

Most people believe in Soul and God, both somehow being part of a higher dimension. Highly intuitive individuals from all cultures tune into this higher dimension. They see "energy" around human beings, called the aura. They speak of energy bodies surrounding the physical body in layers of an etheric, astral, mental and spiritual nature. Science can measure the earth only in plain facts in terms of electromagnetics, but quantum physicists have theories that are compatible with that subtle part of the unmeasurable higher dimension. The mind appears to be capable of transcending time and space; it is part of the fifth dimension. Many of the tools used in what is increasingly being called Energy Medicine are art and are not directly measurable scientifically. We cannot measure directly their effects, but we can measure the results of their effects.

SOME SUBTLE ENERGETIC HEALING PRACTICES

Here are some healing modalities that work with the subtle energetic fields and that I consider to be sacred.

Acupuncture

Acupuncture has been around for approximately 4,000 years. In the last few decades, it has been proven effective in raising ACTH, in treating PMS and male infertility, and in relieving many types of pain. Electroacupuncture, at least when applied to specific acupuncture points that are called the Ring of Fire, is effective in treating diabetic neuropathy, rheumatoid arthritis, depression and migraine headaches, and in raising DHEA (dehydroepiandrosterone). Using Giga frequencies, those in the billions of cycles per second range, Ukrainian physicists and physicians say that they can treat a majority of illnesses as successfully as they can with any drugs, often better—and without complications.

Cranial Electrical Therapy

Cranial electrical therapy with very subtle energy, at one milliampere, a thousandth of an amp of current, can raise beta endorphin and serotonin levels and treat depression and insomnia more safely and better than any drug.

Color and Light

A German physician, Max Lüscher, diagnosed personality and mood with color, accomplishing as much as many of our modern psychometric tests. Phototherapy with various colors influences beta endorphins, melatonin, serotonin and prolactin. Light affects mood, melatonin, serotonin and age of sexual development. The electroencephalogram follows light frequencies. Entrainment, or trance, is easily accomplished with light.

Homeopathy

Two hundred years ago, Samuel Hahnemann developed the concept of homeopathy, the law of similars, using various substances in such highly diluted form that no measurable physical trace remained. Homeopathic physicians report cures of many illnesses. Several modern papers have discussed the effectiveness of homeopathy in treating rheumatoid arthritis, and in our own clinic, we have recently demonstrated that a homeopathic preparation was better than acetaminophen, "the drug doctors prescribe the most for pain."

Sound

Music clearly affects mood. Dr. Alfred A. Tomatis, an otolaryngologist from France, has shown that we cannot speak what we cannot hear. He retrains hearing with sound, and entrainment or trance is easily accomplished with the help of sound. Music therapy is an increasingly popular and successful form of therapy for emotional and physical ailments.

Touch and Healing

Hands-on healing has been proven effective in a statistically significant way. The electroencephalogram can be influenced even by a distant healer. Hemoglobin can be raised by therapeutic touch. DHEA can be raised within minutes by an accomplished spiritual healer.

Aromatherapy

Smell is the most primitive of our senses. Aromas are extremely effective in changing our moods. Recent science demonstrates that even *unsmellable* traces of sweat influence the menstrual cycle of women.

Biofeedback

The Rolls Royce of mind-body medicine, especially when combined with a self-hypnotic technique called autogenic training, biofeedback can control 80 percent of diseases, including high blood pressure and migraines. Psychoneuroimmunology, to some extent, grew out of the initial remarkable findings about biofeedback. Psychoneuroimmunology has provided the aurum potabile ("drinkable gold") for holistic and energy medicine.

All of these techniques, some of which would be considered mind-cure, are a part of sacred healing. From the point of view of the Theist, one who really embraces the sacred as the foundation for all life, the physical body is only a mechanism for work in the physical plane. It is consciousness of the mind and its links with spirit or soul, and through that with God, that can convey reality to the sacred. This consciousness is designed to reflect the qualities and intention of the soul. When human consciousness does not reflect and transmit the qualities and powers of the soul, significant psychological and physical illness can result.

Thus, study of the piano will reveal very little about the nature of sound in general, and certainly the music of the piano will reveal little of the nature of the consciousness of the pianist. A study of the automobile will reveal a bit about the nature of metal and engines but nothing about the driver or the engineers who designed the car. Likewise, the study of the physical in itself will reveal nothing specific about the nature of the spirit or the divine or the sacred. But pragmatic experience reveals that we are endowed with tremendous resources within to heal both physical and emotional problems.

ATTITUDE AND THE NATURE OF THE SACRED

Our state of consciousness, our choice of relation to the divine and the sacred, is under our control. It is ultimately consciousness and our attunement to the divine that determine health, nurturing, love, a desire to do good. A positive, cheerful, optimistic attitude and self-motivation are as important as diet and exercise and, yes, all aspects of modern medicine in determining health and healing.

Consider the following characteristics of a limited human personality and that which we would consider the highest of the spiritual and sacred. Just as common sense will tell you that the column on the right is the wiser choice, so will wisdom allow you to examine the fruits of sacred healing.

The Nature of a Limited Personality	The Nature of the Sacred
negativity	spiritual love
pessimism	joy
materialism	detachment
pride	wisdom
need for authority	abstract thought or reason
desires	intuitive knowing
self-deception	enlightenment
intolerance	acceptance
separatism	unity
cruelty	benevolence
arrogance and selfishness	nobility
prejudice	tolerance
impulsiveness and impatience	peace with serenity
laziness	motivation
destructiveness	cooperation
stubbornness	adaptability responsiveness to spirit
inconsistency of direction	motivation creative purpose
fearfulness	courage
anger, resentment, hatred, jealousy	love and good will
sadness and self-pity	joy
guilt	self-respect

The Nature of a Limited Personality	The Nature of the Sacred
possessiveness	resourcefulness
reactiveness	self-determination
rebellion	harmony and cooperation
greed	charity
sexual profligacy	sexual spiritual attunement
hedonism	productivity and purpose
irresponsibility	responsibility
judgmentalism	discernment
giving up	endurance
ugliness	beauty
untruthfulness	honesty
uncertainty	optimism
annoyance	patience
taking offense easily	dignity
focused on the past	focus on the present

All of these are stressful and involve sympathetic activation, increased adrenalin, a loss of magnesium, exhaustion.

All of these are restorative; parasympathetic, may activate homeostasis effect through subtle quantum well-being.

1

A Physician's
Search for
Sacred Healing

I have always known that there is a universal power we generally call "God," as well as an aspect of us, the soul, that survives physical death.

Although my family was only minimally attached to the concept of going to church, I found the church's rituals comforting and attended regularly throughout my childhood and early adolescence. I grew up attending a Southern Methodist church that was remarkably liberal for its day. Teenagers were allowed to dance on Sunday evenings in the basement of the church. I was not aware of the teachings of guilt that seem so prevalent in many religions today. In my mid-teens I was on a statewide debating team taking the positive side of the debate, "And God so loved the world that He gave His only begotten son that whosoever should believeth in Him would not perish but have everlasting life."

At age sixteen I went off to Duke University where I was often inspired by the sermons of Dr. McClellan, a wonderful Presbyterian minister. Then at nineteen, I entered medical school, three years younger than most of my classmates. I had little time for religion or even thoughts of spirituality over the next eleven years as I pursued medical school, internship, and ultimately a neurosurgical residency at Massachusetts General Hospital. Halfway through the neurosurgical residency, I became engaged, and my fiancé and I discussed at length our spiritual beliefs and what church we would attend. We settled on Trinity Episcopal in Boston, primarily because Dr. Theodore Ferris was one of the most charismatic ministers I've ever encountered. We attended couples' discussion groups at his home about once a month, whenever my schedule allowed.

During post-residency I was still busier with neurosurgery and raising a family than I was with spiritual and religious activity. In October 1971, I founded the first comprehensive pain clinic in the United States. I was dealing with people for whom conventional allopathic medicine had failed. Many of them had undergone multiple, unsuccessful operations. In fact, my average patient had gone through five to seven unsuccessful back operations. Many of them were much worse neurologically and experienced more pain than before the first operation.

In 1972 a synchronous series of events took place. The most important, perhaps, was meeting Olga Worrall, whose work will be discussed at some length later in this book. I had been invited to speak at Stanford University to a group of 1,200 physicians on the value of acupuncture; at that conference I met Olga. I also met Dr. Bill McGarey and subsequently was introduced to the teachings of Edgar Cayce.

Olga and I instantly became friends and remained so for the next thirteen years, throughout the remainder of her life. Through Olga, I was introduced to the concept of "sacred healing." Yes, I was aware that Oral Roberts apparently talked about doing healing on his radio and television programs. My grandmother had been a great fan of his. I was vaguely aware of Katherine Kuhlman and her work in healing. Yet Olga got my attention partly because she had been scientifically studied, and those studies confirmed many unusual abilities and reports of near-miraculous healing.

Knowing how difficult it is to heal many illnesses, especially through neurosurgery, I became fascinated with the idea that miraculous sacred healing could occur. I visited Olga at the Mt. Washington United Methodist Church in

Baltimore, where each Thursday morning about three hundred people attended her healing service at the New Life Clinic.

At the end of August 1972, I visited the Association for Research and Enlightenment (A.R.E.) in Virginia Beach, which houses the Edgar Cayce readings. Edgar Cayce is best known as the "Sleeping Prophet" who did almost 15,000 trance "readings," about two-thirds of them related to illness and healing. "The Week of Attunement," as the conference was called, changed my life even further. Twice I had what is often described as a peak experience, a literal awareness of my connectedness with God and the universe.

Those two events, meeting Olga and the Week of Attunement, led me to the principles and experiences of autogenic training and meditation and finally to a quest for the essence of spirituality. I began collecting letters to Olga from people who claimed she had healed them. Through them I attempted to collect medical documentation to prove sacred healing had occurred as described in these letters. Interestingly, even with the patients' permission, few physicians answered my requests for medical records.

In 1975 I was invited to debate Dr. William Nolen, a surgeon and popular author, on *The Tomorrow Show* with Tom Snyder. Dr. Nolen had written a book titled *Healing:*

A Doctor in Search of a Miracle. Dr. Nolen properly emphasized that healers such as Katherine Kuhlman seemed to feel that many of their cures took place through "the holy spirit." He asserted that many of the illnesses may have been psychosomatic and the results purely the power of suggestion or "placebo."

One case reported in Dr. Nolen's book, however, infuriated me. I knew the patient; he had a pituitary tumor and had lost his ability to see out to the side from either eye. He had been in a hospital in San Francisco and was so distraught after the neurosurgeon there told him all the risks of surgery that he walked out of the hospital in the middle of the night. He went to the Philippines to have "psychic surgery." Two years later, he had totally normal visual fields and no symptoms whatsoever. Dr. Nolen's book, however, gave a different history of this case. On the air I told Dr. Nolen that I thought he had deliberately distorted the facts.

Despite his relatively negative approach toward sacred healing, Dr. Nolen admitted that a significant majority of patients, perhaps as many as 70 percent, were improved by spiritual healers. Yet he concluded his book with "Healers can't cure organic diseases. Physicians can." Then he went on to say, "So let us admit that healers do relieve symptoms and may even, as I've already mentioned, cure some functional diseases." He adds, "We may well admit this; it's a fact—they're going to achieve an overall cure rate of 70 percent."[1] Dr. Nolen's greatest conflict with the sacred healing issue apparently arose from within separate parts of himself!

His statement that he had been "unable to find any such miracle worker"[2] who could cure an incurable illness set me on a course to prove that miraculous healing truly occurred. Over the ensuing years I was able to obtain about twelve medical records documenting such miraculous cures. I wanted at least twenty-five. Now, in the last couple of years, I have been presented with more than one hundred medical records documenting miraculous cures. One white crow proves that there are white crows; we now have a huge flock of them. Sacred healing is alive and well.

THE EFFECTIVENESS OF HOLISTIC HEALING: WHAT'S THE NEXT STEP?

In the meantime, the Shealy Institute that I founded in 1971 continued to work with patients with a wide variety of illnesses. Twenty-six years after its founding, the American Academy of Pain Management, the largest organization of clinical pain practitioners in the world, reported that the

Shealy Institute has the best success of any pain clinic they have evaluated—at a cost that is 60 percent lower than the national average. Our cost effectiveness in dealing with chronic pain of almost every type has been gratifying. When back pain is due to a ruptured disk, we can achieve better and safer results in 85 percent of patients than can be done with surgery. And for those with degenerative joints in the back, 75 percent of the time we can achieve similar results. Seventy-six percent of patients with headaches have a marked reduction in both the frequency and severity of their headaches. This is almost twice as good as any drug on the market. We can get 85 percent of people out of depression with two weeks, safely and without drugs. This also is approximately twice as effective as any antidepressant and without any of the serious side effects.

Yet, what can be done for the 15–20 percent of patients who continue to have chronic pain? And for the patients who come to us with much more serious illnesses, such as cancer? Statistics published in 1997 in the *New England Journal of Medicine* appear to demonstrate that chemotherapy at best might add a few months of longevity to patients with breast cancer, but the quality of life is often markedly diminished.

Another effective healing method needs to be available

for all patients, especially those with medically and surgically incurable illnesses, and those who cannot be cured by the best of alternative medicine. Sacred healing is that method. In this book, I will address the subject of sacred healing and present summaries of cases of documented miraculous sacred healing. And I will demonstrate the physiological effects of sacred healing, including changes in electroencephalogram (EEG), changes in the molecular bonding in water, and other effects, even on bacteria and enzymes.

2

Religion and Sacred Healing through History

From the earliest human times, perhaps 100,000 years ago, when trepanning (the boring of holes into the skull) was performed to let out the evil spirits, healing and religion have been intertwined. According to the *Encyclopedia Britannica*, "Many would hold that the most important function of religion has been that of healing—the diagnosis of the cause of evil and mental and physical sickness, and the development of techniques for its cure." *Britannica* goes on to state, "Rarely can a religious leader succeed unless he can heal; no religion has survived that does not heal."

All great religions include healing in one form or another, ranging from blessings and exorcisms to purification. Ritual formulas, prayers and gestures invoke supernatural power; the power of God can protect the devotee and grant everything from health and fertility to the acquisition of gold. Also, most religions employ charms and amulets, from rosaries to magical mojos, which are blessed in various sacramental ceremonies to perform protective sacred guidance.

In many religions, illness is considered to result from behavioral or moral transgressions. The concept of confession or repentance is common. Religious myths speak of gods, heroes and holy people as healers.

DIVINE ORIGINS OF DISEASE

Many religious traditions have viewed disease as being caused by deities, demons and devils. Exorcism, purgatives, internal cleansing and surgery have been recommended as cures for such predicaments.

Some diseases are associated with loss of soul. A specialty of some shamans, especially among Native Americans, is retrieving human souls. This process is accompanied by meditation, special magical incantations and ceremonies.

Sinning—when an individual has violated a divine law prescribed by his or her religion—has also been viewed as the cause of illness. In this case, curing comes through confession, repentance, enlightenment or the intervention of a holy healer.

The Bible says that King Saul visited a woman at Endor and brought forth Samuel in the spirit who spoke to Saul. Saint Paul, who really founded Christianity, began with a vision of Jesus. Though mediums have undoubtedly existed throughout history, human spiritual mediums appear to have achieved widespread acceptance after 1848.

Spiritualism grew out of this mid-nineteenth-century phenomenon. William James, among others, and Gardner Murphy, the great psychologist from the Menninger Foundation, were members of the American Society for Psychic Research. The various spiritualist organizations, ranging from Spiritual Frontiers Fellowship to the Association of Research Enlightenment, founded by Edgar Cayce and his followers, have emphasized a connection with God and moral principles as the foundation for life. From a spiritualist's perspective, wrong mental (spiritual) thoughts (belief, intent) precipitate disease. The spirit is directly connected with a universal energy called God.

HEALING PRACTICES

Throughout history, the afflicted have sought religious healing in three ways: traveling to a sacred spot (such as one where there is special water to cleanse themselves); consulting a holy person; or obtaining help through a religious object.

Healing Via Water

Springs or temples have typically been the sites to which pilgrimages have been made. Even the Indian vedic tradition states, "The waters are indeed healers; the waters drive away and cure all illnesses."

Water is seen as the source of light both in mythology and science. It is also used in physical and psychological cleansing. Hot springs and mineral waters have long been a feature of spas and health resorts. Evidence from the Neolithic and Bronze Ages indicates interest in such spas in France, Italy, and Switzerland associated with religious and healing traditions. In all, several hundred springs and rivers have been considered to have healing powers.

- In ancient Greece, the springs at Chermoplae and Aedepses were sacred to Heracles.
- In ancient Rome, springs at Tibus and hot sulfur springs at Aquae Abulae were well known.

- In the Middle East, Herod attempted to find relief from his fatal illness at Callirrhoe.
- In ancient Egypt, many of the temples dedicated to the Greek god of medicine, Asclepius, were near or at mineral springs.

The belief that water with healing abilities is charged by a divine presence or a blessing is ancient. Lourdes, in France, is perhaps the world's best-known example. The famous spring achieved its reputation in 1858 after a number of people had visions there of the Virgin Mary. The baths at Scafati, Italy, also contain a shrine to the Madonna. The feast of the Conception of St. John the Baptist is often associated with special healing days. And of course, John baptized people by submersion in water.

From ancient times, a belief has existed in the efficacy of certain rivers in restoring fertility to barren women. Civic, church and private religious healing has taken place at many great rivers. The Euphrates river in Iraq, the Abana and Pharpara in Damascus, the Jordan in Israel, the Tiber in Italy, the Nile in Egypt and the Ganges, Jumna, or Saravati in India have all been associated with purification from transgression, cure of disease and mythical protection into the future.

Healing at Sacred Places

The holy epiphanies are cemeteries or burial places for saints or holy individuals. They are usually surrounded by sacred trees, stones or mountain peaks and are often considered as healing shrines. A good example is the annual pilgrimage to Jerusalem at Easter time undertaken by many Christians. It is interesting that more people go there at the calendar-appointed time of Jesus' death than his birth!

One of the more unusual saints, Saint Rita of Cassea (1381–1456), was reported to have had an incorruptible body. As late as 170 years after her death, Pope Urban XIII viewed the body and reported it to be "as perfect as it had been on the day of her death, with the flesh still of a natural color." About that time, it is reported that her eyes opened and caused a riot! Reportedly, Saint Rita planted a piece of dry wood, watered it each day, and the sticks sprouted into a healthy grapevine, which still bears fruit some 500 years later. The harvest is distributed to high-ranking ecclesiastics. The leaves are dried, made into a powder and sent to the sick around the world. Blessed Antonio Vici (1381–1461) is another of many incorruptible bodies whose burial sites have been reported to have been the scene of miracles of healing.[1]

Holy Healers

A number of monastic orders throughout the world were associated with healing. Some examples are the Knights Hospitalers, the Augustinian Nuns, the Order of the Holy Ghost, the Sorrotes Order and, of course, the Franciscan Order in Europe. Various aspects of the Asclepiads in Greece, the Vomans in India and the Vaidya caste in Bengal also practiced healing. The shamans of many Indian tribes in the Americas have long combined religious and healing practices. Often, healers in indigenous cultures as well as Western civilization trace their knowledge back to the gods.

Perhaps the Franciscan Order has been one of the most successful in maintaining the healing reputation. Many Catholic churches in this country were created by various Franciscan orders of nurses. In the Episcopal church, St. Luke has been the patron saint of hospitals, and of course, the entire Lutheran order has also been much associated with hospitals and healing.

Not only priests, kings and holy people have possessed the abilities to cure. Ordinary individuals have also demonstrated the special power to heal. Sometimes this power comes on spontaneously in a vision; sometimes it has been sought out by the individual through vigorous meditation or mortification of the body. Many great religions were founded by individuals who were believed to have the ability to heal.

There have been many well-known Christian healers in the nineteenth and twentieth centuries. Some of them also founded religions or religious organizations. Among them are John of Kronstadt, Furst zu Hohenlohe-Schillingsfurst, Leslie Weatherhead, Edgar Cayce, Oral Roberts, Kathryn Kuhlman, Phineas Quimby, Mary Baker Eddy, Ernest Holmes and Myrtle and Charles Fillmore.

Mary Baker Eddy founded Christian Science based on Phineas Quimby's work. Quimby, the fountainhead for the entire New Thought Movement, focused on healing, and out of that work came First Christian Science. Then came Unity, founded by Myrtle and Charles Fillmore, and Religious Science, founded by Ernest Holmes. There are subtle but distinct differences in each of these. Essentially, Mary Baker Eddy believed that there was no evil; therefore, there could be no sickness. In Unity and Religious Science, evil and illness or disease are acknowledged, but it is generally believed that one should have a positive attitude and deny the power of evil or the power of the disease over the spirit.

Oral Roberts, at one time a Methodist minister, preached his healing services on radio and television for many years and founded a medical school and hospital in Tulsa,

Oklahoma. Katherine Kuhlman, also at one time active in the mainline Protestant Church, did seminars throughout the country and was accepted even among more fundamentalist churches in Springfield, Missouri. Hundreds of people would attend her ceremonies and often were thrown backwards onto the floor when she touched them.

Perhaps most would not consider him a healer, but Edgar Cayce has had a wider impact in the field than any other modern alternative healer. Cayce went into trances and did almost 15,000 "readings." Two-thirds of these were related to health, and numerous people attested to healings when they applied the recommendations that Cayce made while in trances. The A.R.E. clinic in Phoenix was founded by doctors Gladys and William McGarry, emphasizing many of the principles first proposed by Cayce back in the 1930s and 1940s. My favorite from these has been the use of castor oil, the "Palma Christy," or palm of Christ. It has been demonstrated that a flannel cloth soaked in castor oil and placed on the abdomen with a heating pad will significantly improve immune functions. It is a remarkable palliative treatment for intestinal flu and cramping. Swollen knees also respond extremely well to this particular process, and I have used it both on human patients and on horses for the past twenty-six years.

SPIRITUALITY VS. RELIGION

Perhaps the most important book ever written in the field of religion and spirituality, *The Varieties of Religious Experience*, was written by William James.[2] Born in New York City in 1842, the brother of novelist Henry James, William was educated at Harvard where he also taught from 1872 until 1910. He did classical pioneering work in American psychology and philosophy and was regarded as the leading American philosopher of his time.

Although James admitted, "The field of religion being as wide as this, it is manifestly impossible that I should pretend to cover it," it is interesting that he stated, ". . . the founders of every church owe their power originally to the fact of their direct personal communion with the divine."

The difference between religion and spirituality lies in that statement. Religions tend to establish ritual and dogma to support their particular ideological beliefs. Spirituality is a personal communion with God, soul or divine energy. Of course, religions in their basic philosophy have a great deal in common. These similarities have perhaps best been summarized by Dr. Marcus Bach, one of the great mystics and theologians of this century.

Prayer in the World's Great Religions

CHRISTIANITY:
"When you pray, enter into your closet, and when you have shut the door, pray to your Father which is in secret; and your Father, who sees in secret, shall reward you openly."

CONFUCIANISM:
"Sedulously cultivate the virtue of reverence. When a man is devoted to this virtue, He may pray to Heaven."

BUDDHISM:
"There is no meditation apart from wisdom, and no wisdom apart from meditation. Those in whom wisdom and meditation meet are not far from Nirvana."

HINDUISM:
"I make prayer my inmost friend."

ISLAM:
"Never, Lord, have I prayed to Thee with ill success."

SIKHISM:
"They who cry aloud in trouble obtain rest by prayer and loving God."

JUDAISM:
"Pray to the Lord our God that He may show us the way to go and the thing we should do."

ZOROASTRIANISM:
"He who is called the wise Lord, thou shouldst seek to exalt forever with prayers of piety."

BAHA'I:
"Draw nigh to God and persevere in prayer so that the fire of God's love may glow more luminously in thy heart."

SHINTO:
"If the poorest of mankind come for worship, I will surely grant their heart's desire."

Immortality in the World's Great Religions

JUDAISM:
"The dust returneth to the earth as it was, and the Spirit returneth unto God who gave it."

CHRISTIANITY:
"The gift of God is eternal life, through Jesus Christ our Lord."

ISLAM:
"Those who have believed and done the things which are right, these shall be inmates of Paradise."

JAINISM:
"I know there will be a life hereafter."

CONFUCIANISM:
"All the living must die and, dying, return to the ground, but the Spirit issues forth and is displayed in light."

HINDUISM:
"He becomes immortal who seeks the general good of man."

SIKHISM:
"Why weep when a man dieth, since he is only going home?"

BUDDHISM:
"Earnestness is the path of immortality."

SHINTO:
"Regard Heaven as your father, Earth as your mother, all things as brothers and sisters, and you will enjoy the divine country which excels all others."

TAOISM:
"Life is going forth. Death is a returning home."

ZOROASTRIANISM:
"The soul of the righteous shall be joyful in immortality."

BAHA'I:
"Make mention of Me on earth that in My Heaven I may remember thee."

Peace in the World's Great Religions

CHRISTIANITY:
"Blessed are the peacemakers, for they shall be called the children of God."

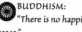 **CONFUCIANISM:**
"Seek to be in harmony with all your neighbors . . . live in peace with your brethren."

BUDDHISM:
"There is no happiness greater than peace."

HINDUISM:
"Without meditation, where is peace? Without peace, where is happiness?"

ISLAM:
"God will guide men to peace. If they will heed Him, He will lead them from the darkness of war to the light of peace."

TAOISM:
"The wise esteem peace and quiet above all else."

SIKHISM:
"Only in the Name of the Lord do we find our peace."

 JUDAISM:
"When a man's ways please the Lord he maketh even his enemies to be at peace with him."

JAINISM:
"All men should live in peace with their fellows. This is the Lord's desire."

ZOROASTRIANISM:
"I will sacrifice to peace, whose breath is friendly."

BAHA'I:
"War is death while peace is life."

SHINTO:
"Let the earth be free from trouble and men live at peace under the protection of the Divine."

Love in the World's Great Religions

CHRISTIANITY:
"Beloved, let us love one another, for love is of God; and everyone that loveth is born of God, and knoweth God. He that loveth not, knoweth not God, for God is love."

CONFUCIANISM:
"To love all men is the greatest benevolence."

BUDDHISM:
"Let a man cultivate towards the whole world a heart of love."

HINDUISM:
"One can best worship the Lord through love."

ISLAM:
"Love is this, that thou shouldst account thyself very little and God very great."

TAOISM:
"Heaven arms with love those it would not see destroyed."

SIKHISM:
"God will regenerate those in whose hearts there is love."

 JUDAISM:
"Thou shalt love the Lord thy God with all thy heart and thy neighbor as thyself."

JAINISM:
"The days are of most profit to him who acts in love."

ZOROASTRIANISM:
"Man is the beloved of the Lord and should love him in return."

BAHA'I:
"Love Me that I may love thee. If thou lovest Me not, My love can no wise reach thee."

SHINTO:
"Love is the representative of the Lord."

Health and Healing in the World's Great Religions

CHRISTIANITY:
"The prayer of faith shall heal the sick, and the Lord shall raise him up."

CONFUCIANISM:
"High mysterious Heaven hath fullest power to heal and bind."

BUDDHISM:
"To keep the body in good health is a duty ... otherwise we shall not be able to keep our mind strong and clear."

HINDUISM:
"Enricher, Healer of disease, be a good friend to us!"

ISLAM:
"The Lord of the worlds created me ... and when I am sick, He healeth me."

TAOISM:
"Pursue a middle course. Thus will you keep a healthy body and a healthy mind."

SIKHISM:
"God is Creator of all, the remover of sickness, the giver of health."

JUDAISM:
"O Lord, my God, I cried to Thee for help and Thou hast healed me."

JAINISM:
"All living beings owe their present state of health to their own Karma."

ZOROASTRIANISM:
"Love endows the sick body of man with firmness and health."

BAHA'I:
"All healing comes from God."

SHINTO:
"Foster a spirit that regards both good and evil as blessings, and the body spontaneously becomes healthy."

The Golden Rule in the World's Great Religions

CHRISTIANITY:
"... All things whatsoever ye would that men should do to you, do ye even so to them .."

CONFUCIANISM:
"Do not unto others what you would not they should do unto you."

BUDDHISM:
"In five ways should a clansman minister to his friends and familiars-by generosity, courtesy and benevolence, by treating them as he treats himself, and by being as good as his word."

HINDUISM:
"Do not to others, which if done to thee, would cause thee pain."

ISLAM:
"No one of you is a believer until he loves for his brother what he loves for himself."

SIKHISM:
"As thou deemest thyself so deem others. Then shalt thou become a partner in heaven."

JUDAISM:
"What is hurtful to yourself, do not to your fellow man."

JAINISM:
"In happiness and suffering, in joy and grief, we should regard all creatures as we regard our own self."

ZOROASTRIANISM:
"That nature only is good when it shall not do unto another whatever is not good for its own self."

TAOISM:
"Regard your neighbor's gain as your own gain and regard your neighbor's loss as your own loss."

NEW THOUGHT AND MIND-CURE RELIGIONS

William James proclaimed that religion is basically a cry for help. To some extent, this cry for help led to what James called the "mind–cure" religions of the New Thought religions: Christian Science, Unity, Religious Science, Divine Science. These churches he considered to be "deliberately optimistic," both speculative and practical.

James felt that the principles of mind–cure came from the New Testament gospels, Emersonian or New England transcendentalism, Berkeleyan idealism, spiritism and Hinduism. Law, progress and development were added to intuitive faith in the healing power of "courage, hope and trust"; "doubt, fear, worry and all nervously precautionary states of mind" were considered harmful.

James went on to state that mind–cure belief had healed blindness, lameness and lifelong invalidism. No less impressive were the moral fruits of positive mind–cure belief. James proclaimed that "deliberate adoption" of positive thinking and cheerfulness led to extensive numbers of individuals achieving "regeneration of character." James mentioned as part of the New Thought mind–cure movement the "Gospel of Relaxation" and the benefit of positive affirmations while going through daily routines.

James considered most mind–cure enthusiasts to be pantheistic (the doctrine that God is the transcendent reality of which the material universe and human beings are only manifestations).[3] Thus this movement incorporated the recently "discovered" Freudian/Jungian subconscious into a concept of intrinsic unity with God, aligning it with transcendental idealism, Hindu Vedantism and Christian mysticism.

James also believed that development of a growing core of love and harmony, emphasizing positivity instead of negativity, led to greater peace and equanimity and freedom from anxiety and tension. He emphasizes the "wonder" of this transformation as the result of simple relaxing.

According to James, religion and spirituality establish "ultimate reality," our private "destiny." Religion provides the zest of life, a sense of peace, and a "preponderance" of love, all of which produce "effects psychological or material" in the physical world.

As ever-expanding scientific technology increased the capabilities of modern medicine, mind–cure brought greater serenity, happiness, and the prevention of certain forms of disease. Both science and New Thought religions led to improvements in health and well-being.

3

The Healer's Role in Medical History

Our knowledge of scientific medicine through the ages has been hampered by poor documentation. Indeed, much has been lost, rediscovered and sometimes lost again.

MEDICINE IN ANCIENT GREECE

We consider Hippocrates (approximately 460–370 B.C.), the best-known Greek healer, to be the Father of Medicine. Even in the time of Hippocrates, it appears that scientists who had the greatest political clout had the most influence on medical beliefs in their areas of expertise. For example, Alcmaeon extensively dissected human bodies. He established the connection between a human's sense organs and the brain. He concluded that the brain serves two purposes: it is the "organ" of the mind responsible for thought and memory, and it is a sensation preceptor. A century later, Aristotle vehemently disagreed with Alcmaeon, declaring the heart to be the center of sensation. Aristotle's theory won out and was accepted for many centuries.

At the time of Hippocrates, the Greeks believed illness could be explained in terms of four basic humors: water, air, fire and earth. Each had corresponding qualities: moist, dry, hot and cold. Basic body fluids were believed to be composed of varying proportions of blood (warm and moist), phlegm (cold and moist), yellow bile (warm and dry) and black bile (cold and dry). Deficiency of these humors would cause diseases. Changes in humors could be caused either by external or internal forces.

Treatment generally consisted of diet, exercise and moderation in such habits as eating, drinking, sleeping and sexual activity. Wounds and sores were cleaned and sprinkled with various herbs. Drugs were taken to induce vomiting. Manipulation was used to reduce dislocations and fractures, and techniques for bandaging were extremely well developed. The Greeks used cautery (singeing of flesh) to treat infections, wounds and tumors, as well as the juice of the opium poppy. As part of the diagnosis, there seems to have been an extensive evaluation of an individual's emotional state, habits, surroundings, behavior and customs.

Some seventy-nine books and fifty-nine treatises make up the *Corpus Hippocraticum*. Though the writings are attributed to Hippocrates, a variety of individuals are believed to have completed the work. Of particular note, the treatises insist physicians should look healthy and be well nourished, to have a "worthy appearance." Decent clothes should be worn, and the healer was directed to exhibit friendliness. Hippocrates is best known for the Hippocratic Oath:

I swear by Apollo Physician and Asclepius and Hygeia and Panacea and all the gods and goddesses, making them my witnesses, that I will fulfill according to my ability and judgement this oath and this covenant:

To hold him who has taught me this art as equal to my parents and to live my life in partnership with him, and if he is in need of money to give him a share of mine, and to regard his offspring as equal to my brothers in male lineage and to teach them this art—if they desire to learn it—without fee in covenants; to give a share perhaps of precepts and oral instruction and all the other learning to my sons and to the sons of him who has instructed me and to pupils who have signed the covenant and have taken an oath according to the medical law, but to no one else.

I will apply dietetic measures for the benefits of the sick according to my ability and judgement; I will keep them from harm and justice.

I will neither give a deadly drug to anybody if asked for it, nor will I make a suggestion to this effect. Similarly I will not give to a woman an abortive remedy. In purity and holiness I will guard my life and my art.

I will not use the knife, not even on sufferers from stone, but will withdraw in favor of such men as are engaged in this work.

Whatever houses I may visit, I will come for the benefit of the sick, remaining free of all intentional injustice, of all mischief, and in particular of sexual relations with both female and male persons, be they free or slaves.

What I may see or hear in the course of the treatment, even outside of the treatment in regard to the life of men, which on no account one must spread abroad, I will keep to myself, holding such things shameful to be spoken about.

If I fulfill this oath and do not violate it, may it be granted to me to enjoy life and art, being honored with fame among all men for all time to come; if I transgress and swear falsely, may the opposite of all this be my lot.

Despite the fact that some American medical schools offer this oath, many aspects of modern medicine are in conflict with it.

The idea of sacred healing appears not to have been a part of Hippocratic medicine. The treatises constantly comment about and devote attention to anatomy in great detail. But no actual spiritual connection is noted.

HEALING IN ANCIENT ROME

The physician Galen (circa 129–200 A.D.) had the greatest influence for about 1,500 years. He reinforced and elaborated on the four fundamental humors mentioned above as the roots of health and illness. Basically, his lasting contribution was to translate the humors into four personalities (phlegmatic, sanguine, choleric and melancholic)—terms still used today. He also dissected extensively, primarily animals and abandoned human corpses. Because he mixed a wide variety of medicinal plants, Galen may deserve recognition as the father of pharmacology.

The introduction of Christianity into the Roman culture gave a strong overlay of religious mysticism to healing. As early as 395 A.D., the Church emphasized healing as being proof of God's grace. Many early hospitals were established by the Church. The Church used numerous icons from early days in healing. Later, various saints and supposedly bits of their bodies or clothes were also used. The emanations or vibrations from these materials could in themselves initiate healing. Many early Christian writers believed disease was cured only through prayer and divine intervention.

Christianity extrapolated based on an earlier Judaic principle that disease equated to punishment for a sin or divine anger. From this religion's beginning, the concept of "the healing mission of Christ" was clearly articulated. In each of the major four gospels of Matthew, Mark, John and Luke (the latter himself a physician), there are numerous instances of Christ acting as a healer in curing paralysis, the inability to speak, blindness, leprosy and fever. Exorcism or "tearing out" of an unclean spirit was also referenced. Throughout the gospels, no clear-cut differentiation exists between faith healing, exorcism and miracles. The means of healing was always considered to be supernatural. Even in those early days, however, touching was extremely important. Christ often reached out to touch the afflicted or allowed them to touch the hem of his garment.

St. Benedict, an early Christian saint, actually forbade the study of medicine. That left the concept of divine healing as the only accepted method for about five hundred years. Surgery and pharmacology regressed during this time. Healing practices consisted of prayer, the laying on of hands, exorcism, amulets of sacred engravings, holy oil, relics of the saints, and very little that would be considered either Hippocratic or scientific.

The concept that holy individuals could have intercessory powers was fully developed during this period. Indeed, proof that an individual was a saint required the performance of healing miracles. Toward the year 1000 A.D. intercessory powers of the Virgin Mary also began to be an important part of the healing ritual. To a large extent, Christian healing ignored the scientific discoveries of Greece and much of the world.

ANCIENT ISLAMIC HEALING

As the Western world was abandoning the principles established in the Greek and early Roman days, the Islamic world markedly improved the pharmaceutical industry by developing such methods as distillation, crystallization, solution supplementation and reduction. Despite these scientific advancements, the Islamic attitude toward the origin of disease remained similar to the Christian idea: Allah caused illness and punished people for their sins. In the Islamic tradition, one could hope for miracles or cures through prayer, and one could also seek divine help through a physician.

Ratzen, a Persian physician and healer, achieved similar recognition in the Arabic/Islamic culture as Hippocrates had done earlier. He wrote approximately 237 books integrating earlier Greek medicine into the Arabic world. A Jewish physician, Maimonides, was another influential healer in the Islam world. Through him and various other Arabic physicians, the condition of hospitals was considerably improved, providing better sanitation, care, facilities and medication than the Western Christian society had accomplished by that time.

THE RENAISSANCE AND HEALING

As the Dark Ages came to an end, medicine began to recover, primarily through the establishment of university medical schools. Until about 1500 A.D., folk healers probably treated a far greater number of patients than did physicians or saints. As the Dark Ages merged into the Reformation, the separation of surgeons from other medical practitioners was virtually completed due to the great disdain for surgery by academic individuals at the time.

The concept of medicine as art and science dominated during the Renaissance, with physicians and artists belonging to the same guild. Perhaps the best-known physician of all was the artist Michelangelo. As was common in those days, individuals often had a broad education and might study medicine but not practice it.

During the Renaissance, the average person was more interested in earthly rewards than heavenly rewards. Gradually, control of hospitals and healing transferred from the Church to the City. Physician training began to be regulated and certified. Ideas of contagion and infectious diseases were organized. Public health institutions were established to care for the hopelessly ill and infirm.

However, physicians were not readily available to the general population. In the thirteenth century in Paris, for instance, only a half-dozen doctors served the public.

Drugs reappeared and were heavily used throughout the Middle Ages, along with digestive assistants such as laxatives, emetics, diuretics, diaphoretics and styptics.

Also, mysticism became widespread. Symbolic procedures, such as chants, were widely used. Astrology was widely recognized. Demons and devils were thought to be common causes of illness, and exorcism by a priest was the only solution. Amulets were commonly used, and various animal parts, especially the genitals, were thought to possess great power.

Attempting to wrest control from the Church and saints, royal healers promoted the concept of the king as the great healer, bestower of the royal touch. Bloodletting, which had been popular even in the earliest days, again became widespread in the Middle Ages.

Perhaps the most famous Renaissance physician was Paracelsus (1493–1541), or Theophrastus Bombastus von Hohenhein. A Swiss physician, he was interested in various mystical and occult sciences and was extremely hostile toward his contemporaries. He believed the influence of the stars and planets upon the "astral body" of the patient was the major cause of disease.

Paracelsus is credited by many for creating modern medicine when he proposed a substitute for the Galen concepts that had dominated for so long. He went back to the *Hippocratic Corpus*. His blending of theological and popular thought integrated mysticism and neoplatonism, and urged a new way of knowing. Jan Baptista van Helmont sought to give form and dimension to Paracelsus' cosmology. During the same period, Frances Baker also established an "alternative path to knowledge of nature."

A French physician, Ambroise Pare, became the leading surgeon of the time. His legacy is his insistence on treating gunshot wounds with boiling oil. Fortunately, he found that it was less efficacious than simple debridement of the wound. He reintroduced cautery and the use of ligatures (tying off) on bleeding blood vessels.

THE SCIENTIFIC REVOLUTION AND HEALING

When the Scientific Revolution began in the 1600s, people started asking *how* instead of *why* things happen. At this time, the major medical treatments were bleeding, purging, dietary restrictions, exercise and the use of various herbs and minerals. Any aberrant mental activity was considered to be "witchcraft." Perhaps the most important drug, quinine, was introduced for the treatment of malaria.

Toward the end of the eighteenth century electricity was introduced, and during much of the nineteenth century various and sundry electrical apparatuses influenced the practice of medicine. (We'll talk more about some of these later.)

The advent of science did much to discourage or displace the earlier practices of sacred healing, the royal touch, laying on of hands, prayer, and so on. Scientific advances in the twentieth century have virtually wiped out reliance on mysticism, saints and sacred healers. Despite this, the failure of drugs and surgery to cure many illnesses, especially chronic ones, has allowed some institutions and "old ways" to remain popular. For example, Lourdes maintains its attraction for those seeking miraculous healing. Folk medicine and various forms of laying on of hands and therapeutic touch continue to be passed down through the ages, enjoying a revival of sorts today.

4

Spirituality and Healing Reawakened

In the June 24, 1996, issue, *Time* magazine reported that 82 percent of the U.S. population believe that prayer can heal, and 77 percent believe in God's intervention in curing serious illnesses. In the April 1997 issue, *USA Weekend* reported that 83 percent of women and 73 percent of men (79 percent of the population) believe spiritual faith can help heal. Fifty-six percent say their faith has helped them heal. Nearly two-thirds of the population (63 percent) believe that doctors should talk to them about their spiritual faith. Today, a spiritual revival is gaining momentum, and sacred healing is reaching its greatest acceptance since the Reformation.

Why this resurgence in a primordial belief that science rejected two hundred years ago? To some extent, it is due to the impersonal nature of modern science and medicine. "Managed care," modern medicine's inadequate answer to financial pressure, is repulsing an increasing number of people. The *very* negative aspects of what I refer to as "Mangled Care" make sacred healing even more attractive and more necessary.

It is also because modern medicine has not fulfilled its promises. Larry Dossey, a respected author and physician, states in his book *Prayer Is Good Medicine* that 80,000 Americans die each year because of infections acquired while in the hospital. This is about twice the number of people killed in automobile accidents a year, more than died in either the Vietnam or Korean wars.

Furthermore, complications from drugs and surgery are the reasons for one-third of patients being admitted to critical care units. "In any other sphere of modern life, this situation would rank as a national scandal," says Dr. Dossey. Compared with prayer, "Modern medicine would win the death derby every time by a landslide."[1]

SACRED HEALING: A VIABLE METHOD TODAY

Dr. William Nolen, in his book *Healing: A Doctor in Search of a Miracle*, stated that healers can cure 70 percent of individuals—a statistic that appears far better than the average drug. Scientific proof indicates that sacred healing is at least as good as most drugs. Virtually no single drug is as effective as sacred healing. Astonishingly, the U.S. Congress, Office of Technological Assessment, has reported 85 percent of the drugs now in use have no satisfactory scientific documentation backing them. Franz Ingelfinger, the late editor of *The New England Journal of Medicine*, once said

> Let us assume that 80 percent of patients have either self-limited disorders or conditions not improvable, even by modern medicine. The physician's actions, unless harmful, will therefore not affect the basic course of such conditions. In slightly over 10 percent of cases, however, medical intervention is dramatically successful. . . . But, alas, in the final 9 percent, give or take a point or two, the doctor may diagnose or treat inadequately, or he may just have bad luck. Whatever the reason, the patient ends up with iatrogenic problems. So the balance of accounts ends up marginally on the positive side of zero.[2]

Although conventional medicine and so-called "scientific" data still diminish the importance of sacred healing's role in medicine, it may be shortsighted to treat it as an orphan or to consider it to be "flaky" or unfounded.

In fact, sacred healing may potentially be one of the

greatest contributions to the health of humanity. I have examined research about the effects of prayer. Also, working with two extraordinary healers, Olga Worrall and Ostad Hadi Parvarandeh, has greatly influenced me. Sacred healing should be the treatment of choice when orthodox medicine has nothing to offer. Ideally, it should also serve as an ancillary treatment of choice even when surgery and drugs are indicated as necessary. As Olga Worrall once said, "Another little touch of healing never hurt anyone." Sacred healing may well be the "aurum potabile" (literally "drinkable gold," meaning gold in solution, which was at one time considered a cure-all) for twenty-first-century medicine.

Sacred healing may hold so much promise because it seems to fulfill the basic laws of nature. Indeed, sacred healing was considered a fundamental part of all healing until so-called "scientific" medicine came along.

To some extent the conflict between materialists and naturalists has existed for at least 2,000 years. Naturalists believe ultimately that human beings cannot create life—that is the province of God. Despite cloning, naturalists would still maintain that we will never create life from inorganic material, and somehow even if we manage to do that, naturalists would assume that it was only because we were working with the "laws" of God and nature. Materialists believe that human beings are the smartest things in the universe and can create anything.

This book presents a concept of the sacred nature of life, spirituality and healing that is more comprehensive than modern physicians have envisioned thus far. Scientific medicine is generally considered to have begun with René Descartes (1596–1650). He wrote the first textbook of physiology, *Treatise of Man*, founded a school of Cartesian physicians, and essentially reconstituted Aristotelian and Galenic thought into his rational dictum. Basically, Descartes introduced the concept that we could understand the whole most completely by breaking it down to its most minute parts and studying them individually. He divorced spirit from life.

One hundred years ago, Sir William Osler, the father of American medicine, wrote, much more eloquently than I can, a philosophy that I believe is even more important today than when he composed it. In addition to diet and exercise, Osler noted the importance of faith in health and healing.

Faith is the great lever of life. Without it, man can do nothing; with it, even with a fragment, as a grain of mustard seed, all things are possible to him. Faith in us, faith in our drugs and methods, is the great stock in trade of the [medical] profession. . . . As Galen says, confidence and hope do more good than physic—'he cures most in whom most are confident.' That strange compound of charlatan and philosopher, Paracelsus, encouraged his patients 'to have a good faith, a strong imagination, and they find the effects.' While we doctors often overlook or are ignorant of our own faith-cures, we are just a bit too sensitive about those performed outside our ranks. We have never had, and cannot expect to have a monopoly in this panacea, which is open to all, free as the sun, in which may make of everyone in certain cases, as was the Lacedemonian of Homer's day, 'a good physician out of Nature's grace.' Faith in the gods or in the saints cures one, faith in little pills another, hypnotic suggestion a third, faith in a plain common doctor a fourth. In all ages the prayer of faith has healed the sick, and the mental attitude of the Suppliant seems to be of more consequence than the powers to which the prayer is addressed. The cures in the temples of Aesculapius, the miracles of the saints, the remarkable cures of those noble men, the Jesuit missionaries, in this country, the modern miracles at Lourdes and at St. Anne de Beaupre in Quebec, and the wonder-workings of the so-called Christian Scientist are often genuine and must be considered in discussing the foundations of therapeutics. We physicians use the same power every day. . . . We enjoy, I say, no monopoly in the faith business. The faith with which we work, the faith, indeed, which is available today in everyday life, has its limitations. It will not raise the dead; it will not put a new eye in the place of a bad one . . . nor will it cure cancer or pneumonia, or knit a bone; but in spite of these nineteenth-century restrictions, such as we find it, faith is a most precious commodity, without which we should be very badly off.[3]

If spiritual healers can assist the belief or faith of a patient, then they may be more important than any drug of surgery! If they can channel Grace, even more so.

Only those patients requiring life- or function-saving medical or surgical intervention (probably no more than 15 percent of patients) need medicine or surgery to help them. Nevertheless, surgery or drug intervention should not be summarily discounted in the cases of serious diseases, such as for major infections, fractures, certain types of cancer curable by surgery or congestive heart failure.

My extremely wise professor of medicine, Eugene A. Stead, Jr., wrote to me in 1978, advising that a physician should primarily serve like a triage officer. When a patient first comes in with a complaint, the role of the physician is to verify that there is no serious illness that requires immediate medical or surgical intervention. If the patient is not suffering from a potentially serious illness, then he or she should be presented with various forms of healing. Indeed, the physician should even consider stepping aside to preclude the patient becoming worse off.

Drugs and surgery are inappropriate for many chronic illnesses, especially those representing stress reactions without measurable physical dysfunction. This is most true for depression, anxiety and panic attacks, and all of the psychoneurotic and neurotic illnesses. Even for chronic illnesses, where drug therapy could improve quality of life for diabetes or congestive heart failure patients, it is always appropriate to complement or supplement those therapies with a safe alternative. For instance, insulin certainly may be required in diabetes, but the addition of chromium picolinate, 1000 micrograms per day, and vanadium 50–100 micrograms per day, might enable a patient who develops diabetes after age thirty-five to reach a point where insulin isn't needed. And there is certainly some evidence in some patients that sacred healing could assist in diabetes.

Potentially beneficial alternatives to consider may

include acupuncture, transcutaneous electrical nerve stimulation, hypnosis, biofeedback, creative imagery, osteopathic manipulative therapy, chiropractic therapy, improved nutrition, Reiki therapeutic touch, massage, homeopathy, light and color therapy and aromatherapy. In a sense, all these approaches are part of the divine and sacred. All of these alternatives are described in *The Complete Family Guide to Alternative Medicine* (Element Books, 1996) for which I was a consulting editor. No one modality is a cure-all for all illness. Judgment of the therapist and belief of the patient probably should determine which alternative approach is appropriate in a given situation.

5

Outstanding
Healers
of Our Time

I have been open to sacred healing for some twenty-five years. But just as there appear to be very few outstanding intuitive diagnosticians at this time, there are very few outstanding healers. We will discuss a few of them in detail in this chapter.

If sacred healing is to be a significant factor in the future of medicine, it appears to me that formal testing of these individuals' healing abilities needs to be done. If sacred healing is to be of value, we need many more sacred healers, especially those who have demonstrated their ability in a way that is scientifically documentable.

There is still no standard scientific testing of the ability of a healer to heal. Many individuals call themselves healers; many of them may achieve results through the placebo or faith aspect of their patients. In the long run, however, it is documentation of healing otherwise physically "incurable" diseases, those not curable by drugs or surgery, that really proves the efficacy of a healer.

I believe that 85 percent of physicians go into medicine because of their compassion and altruistic desire to help patients. Most of them are healers in the true sense of the word. Yet modern medicine has done little to increase longevity and perhaps even less to enhance the quality of life. Thomas McKeown, the British professor of social medicine, brought to our attention that only 8 percent of the longevity gain in the twentieth century can be attributed to the "miracles" of modern science. Instead, pasteurization of milk, chlorination of water, improved sewage control and better nutrition have contributed the remaining 92 percent gain.

HARRY EDWARDS, FOREMOST ENGLISH HEALER

Harry Edwards, probably the best-known sacred healer in England and former president of the National Federation of Spiritual Healers, believes that anyone with a great passion and desire to help others can develop the ability to heal. Sally Hammonds reported that Edwards is a very humble man who seemed free of ego, despite his strong beliefs in spiritualism and healing. Edwards has been quoted as saying the qualifications of a good healer include generosity, a willingness to give of self, compassion and sympathy for those in need. He feels that individuals who want payment for their healing are too selfish and, therefore, not as likely to be outstanding healers.

In the mid-1970s, Edwards was receiving up to 9,000 letters a week from patients requesting absent healing. Today, Edwards holds a universal absent healing moment at ten o'clock GMT each night. English viewers can tune in and join Edwards in his healing moment.

Although Edwards is a gifted healer, Sally Hammonds reported that most people had to return to him for treatment a number of times. A single healing experience rarely cured people of their disorders. He also encouraged patients to help themselves. In treating chronic arthritic conditions, for instance, Edwards recommended home massage and specific limbering exercises, in addition to multiple laying-on-of-hands sessions. He feels a patient's mind has to be influenced toward healing. Edwards believes that mental distress is caused by emotional and sexual problems, failure to attain one's ideals, and the desire of the inner self to express in a way that the existing way of life does not permit.

Edwards particularly emphasizes positive thinking to overcome negativity. Despite the importance he places on divine energy in healing, Edwards feels atheists can be healed. He reports that 80 percent of his patients improve from his treatments and belief system; 30 percent are cured; 10 percent are cured instantly.

OLGA WORRALL: THE MOST STUDIED HEALER OF ALL TIME

I first met Olga Worrall in 1972 at a meeting about acupuncture at Stanford University in California. Her husband Ambrose had died the previous year. Olga had continued her healing services at the Mount Washington United Methodist Church in Baltimore, Maryland, where the two of them had worked together for almost thirty-five years. Olga conducted healing services, with about 300 attendees, every Thursday morning. It appeared to me that most attendees at the Mt. Washington United Methodist Church were repeat visitors.

Olga stated that the healing service "exhilarates me. I feel seven feet tall. I'm just a channel for the healing power, but the power comes from spiritual sources, not from me." She had thousands of letters in her possession from people attesting to her healing powers. Many of these cases were difficult to assess from a medical point of view. The accounts described illnesses that could not be easily measured, such as anxiety, difficulty in breathing and many symptoms that are not exactly medical diagnoses.

Typical of the thousands of letters received by Olga Worrall—and we now have more than 15,000 of these—are the following:

- A fifty-two-year-old woman writes: "During the service I felt heat moving throughout my body. My dizziness disappeared completely, and I have remained free of it now in the months since the healing service."
- Another letter states: "My arthritis pain which had been virtually incapacitating for the last year has been almost totally absent since last Thursday morning. Praise God."

More than a hundred cases could be followed up for medical proof that these patients were indeed cured. I wrote to patients personally, asking permission to contact their physicians for medical records. All of the patients gave me permission. When I wrote to the physicians, however, the vast majority never acknowledged my letters. I finally obtained medical records for nine patients who could be considered to have been miraculously cured of a variety of illnesses.

The findings of Dr. Elmer Green and his wife Alyce, psychology researchers from the Menninger Foundation who tested Olga, were perhaps the most startling. The Greens visited me in LaCrosse, Wisconsin, in September 1977. Olga was connected to various electrical monitoring equipment, including EEG, EKG, skin electrical potential, temperature and so on. She was placed in a room that had a vacant room on either side of it. Two more rooms along the hallway on the opposite sides of the vacant rooms were used. One was for recording the measurements during the study, the central control room. The other one, four rooms away, on the other side of the second vacant room, held the patient, wired in a similar way to Olga.

Olga could not see the patients she was treating, nor had she been introduced to them or informed about their problems. Her voice was recorded into the central control room, as were the physiologic monitoring from both her and the patient. In four out of the twelve patients, there were striking simultaneous EEG changes associated with the exact moment during which Olga "sent" healing. When working with one patient, she stated, "I believe this patient smokes, as it feels as if I'm moving through molasses to get my energy to him." She was right.

Although I could write books about Olga, two final quotes from this great healer are most notable. Olga said back in the early 1970s, "One form of cancer in particular is a viral disease. . . . The mycin drugs often trigger cancers, too, by disturbing the blood chemistry of the body."[1] She said she had been told about that in the 1950s.

OTHER NOTABLE MODERN HEALERS

Today there are a number of healers in this country who appear to achieve some remarkable results, although I have no medical documentation for most of them.

Ron Roth, a former Catholic priest, sent me many letters from patients who considered themselves healed. When I tried to verify them, the situation was the same as with Olga's letters. Physicians simply are unwilling to provide records, even when a patient permits it. Three proofs of miraculous healing, however, were obtained from Roth's group of patients.

The work of Sister Justice Smith, a professor at Rosary Hill College in Buffalo, New York, has been of great importance. She found that Mr. Esterbane, a healer studied extensively in the late 1960s and early 1970s by Dr. Bernard Grad, in Canada, could (as did Olga) "heal" trypsin, an enzyme that breaks down protein when the trypsin had been extremely damaged mechanically. Dr. Grad also demonstrated remarkable healing by Mr. Esterbane of controlled-size skin wounds on rats.

Miatek Wirkus, formerly of Poland and now living in Maryland near Washington D.C., has an outstanding reputation as a healer in this country. I have "proof" of his ability to heal some individuals with severe hearing loss. Markedly improved audiograms in six patients are impressive.[2]

Ethel Deloach and Ethel Lombardi are other American healers of repute. Although I do not have any personal records of their healings, they speak widely and are considered very reputable among alternative healers.

One of the more unusual healers that I had an opportunity to meet and evaluate briefly is Reverend Bill Brown, originally a Presbyterian minister who became an "etheric surgeon." In the mid-1970s, I visited Brown in Georgia and observed his healing. He also treated my own neck problem.

Brown went into a very deep trance. Without actually touching my body, he went through motions as if injecting anesthesia, as well as various surgical maneuvers. His hands turned deep, almost beet red and were extremely warm. Unfortunately I had no thermistors with me to measure the temperatures, which may have been well above his body temperature. (Although Brown verbally reported many cures, I was never able to obtain medical records attesting to his ability to heal.)

A young Russian, Boris Parfenov, is twenty-four years of age. In five of six situations he was quite capable of affecting the EEG from a distance of one hundred feet and on five occasions from a distance of 160 miles. These changes do not unequivocally prove that healing is occurring, but they certainly show a remarkable influence of a healer from a distance.

Recently I met Richard Gordon, who developed a technique that he calls Quantum Touch. The principles of Quantum Touch as outlined by Gordon are

1. Energy follows thought—practitioner uses intention and various meditations to raise and move the energy.
2. Breathing amplifies the Life-Force.
3. The practitioner raises his or her vibration to create a high-energy field and uses that field to surround the area to be healed.
4. Resonance and entrainment cause the area being

healed to change vibration to match that of practitioner. The practitioner simply raises and holds the new resonance.

5. No one can really heal anyone else. The person in need of healing *is* the healer. The practitioner simply holds a resonance so that can happen.

6. The energy follows the body-intelligence to do the necessary healing. The practitioner pays attention to body-intelligence and "chases the pain."

7. When energy moves through a blockage, it causes heat both in the practitioner and the patient.

8. The practitioner is also getting a healing by doing the work.

9. The ability to assist in healing is natural to all people.

10. Quantum Touch works well when combined with all other healing modalities.

11. Trust the Process. The work may cause temporary pain or other distressing symptoms that are all part of the healing. The Life-Force and the healing process work with a complexity and wisdom that are beyond our conception.

When Mr. Gordon visited us, he taught four people on our staff his technique, which consists of centering one's mind, detaching from all concerned, entering essentially a quiet meditative state, and beginning to feel one's own internal energy, chi, qi, or prana, moving from the legs up and out through the hands or fingers. Once one has this internal sensory process going, then the Quantum Touch therapist applies his or her hands near or around the areas where patients have difficulties. It may be to any part of the body from the top of the head to the tips of the toes. We also had Mr. Gordon "apply" his Quantum Touch principles without touching the patient's body, and in three out of three situations he was clearly capable of altering the EEG during his "sending" of energy to the patient.

As a result of the meeting at the A.R.E. in Virginia Beach in 1972, I also developed a profound interest in intuitive diagnosis. I have been fortunate to study and work with several remarkably talented intuitive diagnosticians, particularly Dr. Robert Leichtman and Dr. Caroline M. Myss. For the last seven years Caroline and I have been teaching a course in intuition. Increasingly, I receive requests for validation from people who claim to be medically intuitive; a few have great talent. Undoubtedly, in the near future, it will be necessary for us to establish programs to train and authenticate those individuals who truly have medical intuitive capabilities.

PSYCHIC SURGEONS

"Psychic surgery" is done primarily in the Philippines and Brazil. In September 1976, I was a participant in a team (with the Greens, another physician, and a film crew) that visited seven psychic surgeons in the Philippines who perform surgery without tools other than their minds and hands. Six of the healers produced what appeared to be blood on the surface of the skin of their patients during the psychic surgery. I was able to take those blood samples from twenty-two of the patients by swabbing with cotton. All the samples proved later to be human blood.

I saw three specific types of psychic surgeons. Two individuals went into deep trances. Their eyes rolled up into their heads and fluttered as they worked. More commonly the healer did not seem to go into a trance and could carry on a perfectly normal conversation with us during the healing process.

One of these psychic surgeons, Tony Santiago, treated a male patient whose bladder cancer was significant enough to be seen through his thin skin. As Santiago placed his hands on the patient's abdomen, liquid blood and blood clots about the size of small popcorn popped out and splattered all over the room. I was able to collect a number of these clots, and they indeed were human blood. However, the size of the tumor did not change visibly.

There were two cameras focused on Santiago and three scientific observers watching. It was quite clear there was no sleight of hand. Santiago's pulse escalated to about 135 beats per second at the height of his healing.

Tony Agpaou, at that time the best-known healer in the Philippines, said to me, "You know, Norman, we only do these materializations because they give the patients faith in our ability." With that, he moved his hands about a foot apart and held them over the abdomen of a woman who did not speak English. As I looked down, it seemed as if her abdomen were opening, revealing the peritoneum, a shiny transparent membrane inside the abdomen and covering the organs. I could even see what looked like omentum, a fatty layer, through the peritoneum. I got down on my knees. The image I was seeing was at least a centimeter above her abdomen, not even touching it. Without moving his hands, Agpaou said, "And, just as we can materialize, we can dematerialize." The image then disappeared.

On a number of occasions over the course of an entire day, Agpaou materialized not only liquid blood but sometimes blood clots and at times bits of white tissue that looked like fascia, which is the substance between tissue planes within the body. He had on a short-sleeved shirt that could not hide anything. I followed him around, even going into the bathroom with him. I was allowed to look under the top of the table and in drawers in the room where he worked. He probably "produced" three pints of blood from various patients treated during that day.

One of the most interesting healers in the Philippines, known as Padre Tierte, worked in a small sanctuary where we witnessed him removing blood and some evidence of magnetic healing. He also removed some foul-smelling material, more than a pint in volume, from a woman's back. Smelling like the worst kind of rotting marsh, it is hard to believe something like that could have been hidden in the room. The aroma was so strong that I almost vomited when it appeared.

A fascinating event occurred when Jun Labou worked on Alan Neuman, the producer/director of the television program that was being filmed during our trip. Labou told Neuman that he had mucus on his heart. Working primarily on Neuman's neck, Labou placed his hands deep between the trachea and the sternocleidomastoid muscle. Out poured at least several ounces of pure pus. He massaged the skin over the upper chest and more pus came out of Neuman, then at the end a few drops of blood. It looked very much as if an abscess had been opened by a surgeon's knife. I obtained samples of this, and it proved to be pus with many white blood cells present. I do not know any way in which pus can be stored and produced on call, with a few drops of blood then appearing, as happens when an abscess under pressure is opened. It is difficult to be certain that any healing took place as there was no medical evaluation earlier.

A year after our visit to the Philippines, Jun Labou was brought to our clinic (at that time in LaCrosse, Wisconsin), where he performed psychic surgical procedures on seventeen patients. Again, blood appeared. I was able to obtain samples of blood from two of the patients, as well as the blood that Labou removed. Also, I obtained a sample of Labou's blood. A forensic pathologist in Berkeley, California, who examined the samples assured me that in each case the blood was that particular patient's blood type and not Jun Labou's blood.

During these procedures, I never personally saw a patient's skin actually open. It was always as if the blood were welling up, as if it were coming through the skin. Some Brazilian and Philippine films of psychic surgery do show possible openings of the skin; however, no scar or evidence of the procedure is visible on the patient's skin at the conclusion of the procedure.

THE IMPORTANCE OF ATTITUDE

A healer from New Zealand has worked on a number of patients at our clinic on several occasions. Rod Campbell is also an author. He says, "The people who have permanent recoveries, even after being told there was nothing medical science could do for them, are the people who have a complete change of attitude. After being told they have a very short time to live, they then see and appreciate the little things they never had time to see before."[3]

Rod gives a number of case histories and reports of healing patients. I think some of his remarks on his experiences are particularly noteworthy.

I have found it is necessary for me to keep my mind on the fact that the energy is coming from God. Prayer can assist in keeping the minds of the healer and patient on the fact that the energy is coming from God.

The gift of healing is to glorify God, so if we're willing to accept his healing it seems right that we give thanks to him while we are making use of his gift.

[In response to the question, what is the role of the healer, and why can't the angels do it on their own?]

The only reason seems to be that God wants us to have love and respect for each other . . . then we will also come to have love and respect for all living things and all he created.

If you do have sympathy, love, and respect for someone suffering, and you would like to make things easier for them, please try.

While Dr. Wilson of the Foundation for the Study of Subtle Energies was doing his research, he found some were losing their ability when their ego or the dollar sign came into their minds.

Unfortunately, even when the healer does everything right, the patient must have a change in attitude for the healing to be effective.

Other people's influences can allow the patient to turn back and recreate their [sic] diseases. No amount of healing will be permanent if this is happening.

Edgar Cayce's Emphasis on the Importance of State of Mind

Although Edgar Cayce was not a healer in the usual sense, he did almost 10,000 trance readings related to health and illness. Scores of books have been written about his work. Cayce emphasizes that *all* healing ultimately is spiritual, involving atonement with God or a divine force, assisted by the patient's attitude, by physicians of various persuasions or by prayer or sacred healers. His most frequent spiritual message was

Know that all strength, all healing of every nature is the changing of the vibrations from within—the attuning of the Divine within the living tissue of a body to Creative Energies. This alone is healing. Whether it is accomplished by the use of drugs, the knife, or whatnot, it is the attuning of the atomic structure of the living cellular force to its spiritual heritage. (Cayce reading 167-1, M.24, 7/25/39)

Other observations from his readings:

• But if your mind holds to it, and you've got a stumped toe, it will stay stumped. If you've got a bad condition in your gizzard, or liver, you'll keep it if you think so. (Cayce reading 257-249, M.49, 12/5/42)
• Medications only attune or accord a body for the proper reactions from the elemental forces of divinity within each corpuscle, each cell, each activity of every atom of the body itself. (Cayce 1173-6, M.28, 1/14/36)
• [N]o mechanical appliance does the healing. It only

attunes the body to a perfect coordination and the Divine gives the healing. For life is divine, and each atom in a body that becomes cut off by disease, distrust or an injury, then only needs awakening to its necessity of coordination, cooperation with the other portions that are divine, to fulfill the purpose which the body, the soul, came into being. (Cayce 1173-7, M.28, 11/28/36)

- Thus does spiritual or psychic influence of body upon body bring healing to any individual; when another body may raise that necessary influence in the hormone of the circulatory forces as to take from that within itself to revivify or resuscitate diseased, disordered or distressed conditions within a body. (Cayce 281-24, Prayer Group Series, 6/29/35)

OSTAD HADI PARVARANDEH: A GRAND MASTER HEALER

Despite having worked with many healers, until meeting Ostad Hadi Parvarandeh, I had documented medically miraculous healing in less than a dozen patients. Ostad's healing abilities, as this book demonstrates, are truly remarkable.

By his own account, Ostad's childhood was normal.

Born in Tehran, Iran, on May 13, 1926, Ostad was the second of five children. His father was an administrator at the American University in the Department of Education in Tehran. Ostad says his father had "a little bit" of ability to heal. (His father's touch could alleviate pain.) He describes his mother, who lived to be 89, as a homemaker.

Ostad is convinced his ability to heal has been nurtured by his intense attention to God from early childhood. The Parvarandeh family was spiritually oriented, and he had a religious upbringing. It was very hot in the summertime where he grew up, so he often chose to sleep on the roof of the family's home. While nodding off, he would study the bright stars in the sky, thinking a great deal about God and the creation of the earth.

Ostad saw a lot of his grandparents. One grandmother lived with them, and his first healing experience involved this grandmother. She had a ongoing physical problem, which appears to have been *tic douloureux* (a painful tic). When Ostad was seventeen or eighteen years old, his grandmother had a severe attack. While she was in great pain, he happened to touch her, and the pain immediately disappeared.

About that time, a neighbor invited Ostad to accompany her on a hospital visit to see a patient she knew. He went along to please her. Two days later, the same neighbor asked him again to go, and he did. The third time she asked, Ostad said he did not wish to go because he really did not know the patient that well. Nevertheless, the neighbor prevailed, saying the patient had no family. The real reason, however, was that the patient felt so much better when Ostad was there that his presence had been requested.

At first, Ostad wondered whether his eyes might be the source of his healing power. Even as a child he could hypnotize. Later, he hypnotized people to get them to divulge a wide variety of information.

One instance of this occurred when a brother-in-law had disappeared and his sister wanted to learn his whereabouts. During World War II, the brother-in-law had deliberated whether to go to Russia and involve himself in the war effort. Ostad hypnotized his other sister, the one not married to this man. In her trance, she told him the brother-in-law was located in a small room in another city. She described the room's location with such detail that Ostad and his married sister visited the house described and knocked on the door. He was there.

Though very good at hypnotizing, eventually Ostad decided it was not a wise practice. He was concerned about possible loss of control. During the next few years, when he was in his late teens, he was asked often to heal people's headaches and other pains, but he did so only sporadically and not as a driving avocation.

Ostad chose to attend the American University in Tehran and graduated with majors in French and English. Because of his skills in these languages, he became an Iranian diplomatic counsel to France. Over the next few decades, he served in a number of countries, including Greece, Yugoslavia, and Bulgaria before retiring in 1976.

Early in his career, Ostad became politically involved in the Iran/American Society, where he met his wife, Fari. Theirs has been a very happy marriage. Ostad and Fari have two grown sons and grandchildren who also live in the United States.

During his governmental service, Ostad restricted his healing, seeing perhaps two or three people a day. Following retirement, his healing ministry really began. His home practically became a clinic. At times, so many people gathered outside the house requesting his attention that police had to assist with traffic control. His hours were from 7:00 A.M. to 7:00 P.M. and occasionally until 10:00 P.M. His following was so large he could hardly leave home without people begging for his attention.

Despite the healing load Ostad was carrying, he found

time to train twelve physicians and eight assistants to heal using his techniques. Ostad says many of them are quite good at it, but none can match his capability for healing serious illnesses. He recognizes his own powers as being innovative and unique.

Ostad is well acquainted with medical terminology. I believe this has come about through solving thousands of patients' problems, sometimes more than a hundred people a day, and through his association with his physician brother. He also refers to "the big computer in the sky" to which he has access. As years have passed, his ability to diagnose a situation has became even more acute.

Since 1976, Ostad has used a set of beads and other objects as pendulums to help in finding answers for healing. While swinging these tools gently, he concentrates on the problem to be solved, asking himself questions: "What is the nature of this person's disease?" "Might it be cancer, or a kidney or liver problem?" "Are nerves involved, or is it muscle difficulties?" Often he gets information "in my mind," whereas sometimes his pendulum is the medium. He ultimately refines his questioning in each situation to the point where he asks himself whether a specific hormone (for example, FSH, LH or oxytocin) might be the problem.

Since childhood, Ostad has also been able to see a person's physical aura, both its color and movement. He believes disturbances in an individual's energy show areas of illness. All illnesses are associated with a dark color or discoloration in the energy field and an error in the normal pattern of circulation of this energy.

Interestingly, as soon as Ostad tunes in to patients, he believes he can also tell the types of diseases that plagued their mothers or fathers. To diagnose patients' problems, he views the energetic connection between the patients and their parents.

Basically, Ostad believes that organ dysfunctions cause most diseases. Infections from bacteria outside the body are rarely the cause of a disease. Ostad says every organ in the body is connected to all others, which is certainly energetically and physiologically correct, but he has a specific concept about the "duties" of the organs. For instance, he says heart disease results from the pancreas not functioning properly. When it is functioning normally, no blood vessels will block the heart. This makes sense to me because the pancreas must have adequate lipase to influence fat metabolism.

According to Ostad, a mental disease or a major brain dysfunction is an impossibility when the adrenal glands are functioning normally. In other words, the adrenal glands, when adversely influenced by anger, for example, can affect the mind or brain.

Ostad believes certain crystals, pyramids, acupuncture, music, types of electricity and electromagnetic stimulators may assist with healing. But he thinks sacred healing is superior.

A healer can transfer his or her energy to other materials, usually something edible, such as water, raisins or sugar. The patient may then use the food to reinforce healing.

I have observed Ostad using energized materials while healing. He commonly gives an energized sugar cube or raisins to a patient with whom he is working. He tells the patient to bite off a few grains of the sugar cube or eat a raisin at intervals. Each time, the patient is asked to repeat: "In the name of the most merciful God." The statement reinforces the healing Ostad sets in motion.

When Ostad uses energized water, he has the patient sip the water to assist in the healing process. Ostad also "charges" iron, zinc and lead to make them more useful in the body or less toxic, as the case may be. Ostad energizes herbs, vitamins, food substances and so forth, to enhance their benefits. He carefully selects the energized material for each patient, determining whether a given food is useful or might be harmful.

He has no opposition to certain drugs prescribed by physicians when used under certain circumstances. However, he thinks a master healer should determine whether a drug may be useful to the patient.

Besides continuing his healing practice, Ostad had a new mission when I met him. As a master healer, his lasting contribution would be to document comprehensively his findings concerning disease sources. Also, he intended to train talented individuals to carry on his life's work of sacred healing. He wanted to world to know about the external toxins, lifestyles and personal consciousness that affect our health and well-being.

In addition to information Ostad conveyed to his students while in their physical presence, the students say Ostad visits them in their dreams. He imparts further information to them and sometimes suggests which questions they should be asking him. In other words, the association between teacher and student becomes a very close spiritual connection.

The master healer believes the soul is a part of overall divinity. Divine energy cannot be measured, and it is different from electromagnetic energy. Divine energy travels instantly through time and space and can be directed by such talented individuals.

THE CHARACTERISTICS OF
A MASTER HEALER[4]

Why can a healer transmit energy while a regular person cannot? A master healer's mental attitude and life of prayer and devotion produce a more direct connection with divine energy. For this reason a healer can tap into divine energy much more effectively than individuals who do not have spiritual practices. A master healer pays continuous attention to and is totally devoted to God. To heal, the healer must continuously be in touch with God, maintaining a constant mental and spiritual connectedness.

Ostad emphasizes that prayer and meditation improve one's energy field. He uses the example of astral travel. Individuals who are not truly in tune with the divine cannot do astral travel. However, the process can be learned through practice with prayer and meditation. He sees the astral energy body, if you will, as a protective mechanism for a human being.

Ostad, whose own religion is Islam, respects all religious beliefs, though he does not believe in reincarnation. He says, "The Creator is not running short of creation! Everyone lives only once on earth." When pressed, Ostad says, "Jesus Christ was a great prophet, as was Mohammed. They're all

part of the center of God. Both were great prophets in different times serving different people." He considers God to
be the totality of the universe; everything represents God.

Cosmic Energy

Every atom in the body is basically in touch with cosmic or
divine energy, and each body has its own individual and
unique cosmos. This is certainly apparent from an electromagnetic perspective. We are all electromagnetic entities.
Ostad believes that divine energy makes us more unique
than our obvious physical and personality traits do. Each of
us has a unique individual energy influenced by the soul that
is in contact with the divine. Energy circulates throughout
the universe, with a particular pattern of energetic connectedness between an individual and the divine.

Clairvoyants are able to see angels around a master
healer when that person is healing. Authentic clairvoyants
report seeing changes in the healer's energy field during
healing sessions.

Ostad emphasizes the importance of a true healer being
very closely connected with God. This means living a life
free of behavior that is not sacred. He feels that a person
who drinks, smokes or partakes in a lascivious lifestyle
cannot be a good healer. Under no circumstances will a

healer use drugs or alcohol or get angry. To have continuous access to divine energy, the healer must be virtuous and pure in heart.

The healer provides a much more comprehensive and holistic overview of a disease than modern medicine, which tends to identify a single cause. A master healer looks at the entire person to understand disease at its most fundamental physiological nature, whether it originated in the red cells, the white cells, the platelets, or because of some other malfunction or toxicity. (These concepts are unique to Ostad's belief system.)

Although a healer should not get rich by healing, Ostad believes in a healer's right to earn a living from his or her work. Ostad says under ordinary circumstances a healer volunteers healing but can request donations. Attitudes of humbleness and mission are important. We have trouble understanding these criteria in the United States.

HOW DOES A HEALER HEAL?

A true healer need not be present in the room or even in the vicinity of a patient. Ostad can heal a patient residing in London, England, while he is in San Francisco, California. Healing from a distance occurs at a speed faster than light, essentially faster than what we would think of as time. The implication here is that time and distance play no part in a master healer's effect on a patient.

A master healer can diagnose what is wrong with an individual by hearing the patient's voice on a tape or over a telephone, by seeing a photograph, preferably of the entire front and back of the body, or by knowing the full name of the individual. A diagnosis will include all known diseases but sometimes will give information about a disease that's not known to physicians.

Once Ostad trusts an individual who is closely associated with the patient, such as a daughter caring for a parent or one of his students, he is able to convey his ability to that individual, even across distances. The representatives are then able to perform certain healing techniques or healing of specific diseases. The healer can grant permission to others to tap into his or her energy bank.

With the healer's permission, students or others are able to see and feel the energy systems and the auras of other individuals. A master healer can also change both his or her own aura and the aura of others.

Ostad sees many different forms of energy that may be channeled for healing. These may take the shape of rain, a wave, a tornado, a bullet, a spiral or a laser. Furthermore, specific colors are associated with healing energy, just as there are specific colors associated with the health of the energy of one's body, or the chakras. The colors generally are turquoise or green, sometimes pink and sometimes golden. All of these are associated with health. Dark colors, browns, black or smudgy colors that are not distinctly clear are associated with illness. These do seem to vary tremendously from individual to individual.

The intent of the healer is the dominant factor. The healer must pay attention in order to control the transfer of healing or divine energy either locally or remotely.

A master healer does not catch the patient's illness during the healing session. Furthermore, the healer does not have to muster his or her own energy to heal. An authentic healer never loses energy and is never fatigued or de-energized during the process.

A master healer both sees auras and feels the patient's energy. Seeing energy refers to both an individual's electromagnetic energy field and divine energy.

According to Ostad, Einstein's theory ($E = MC^2$) is perfectly reflected in the healing process. The healer is able to convert mass into energy. For example, the dissolution of a cyst or tumor would be converting mass into energy. Conversion of energy into mass would be the regeneration of tissues, such as in a cirrhosis cure.

The Chakras

The chakras or energy centers in the body are focused on in many healing modalities. When the chakras are unbalanced or blocked, illness can occur. Ostad recognizes only five chakras (many healers work with seven or more):

1. The third eye chakra, which controls the entire body;
2. The heart chakra, which strengthens the entire body and works with the brain in influencing clairvoyance. It is not, he says, associated with love as traditionalists claim;
3. The liver chakra, which also strengthens the entire body;
4. The spleen chakra, which decreases pain and controls the manufacture and functioning of blood cells;
5. The navel chakra, which affects sexual functioning and love.

Ostad thinks individual organs also influence well-being. For instance, the adrenal gland is responsible for and involved in emotions such as anger, depression and anxiety. The brain generally controls all organs in the body.

6

Spirituality, the Basis for Healing

In the last thirty years America has gone from believing "God is Dead" to embracing spirituality, at least in the media's opinion. Yet several common beliefs seem constant throughout the last fifty years. Back in the 1940s, Carl Jung, the great Swiss psychiatrist, studied people around the world and reported that approximately 90 percent of individuals in virtually all cultures believe in

- life after death (a soul);
- a supreme being (God);
- the Golden Rule (Treat thy neighbor as thyself).

Jung stated that people who do not share the age-old beliefs listed above do not thrive. The existential crisis of doubt about purpose or spiritual meaning in life may be a major root cause of many illnesses.

Evelyn Underhill, a great Christian mystic, stated that spirituality is not living in a monastery or nunnery. It is the *attitude* you hold in your mind when down on your knees scrubbing the steps.[1] Indeed, it is the right approach to life whether engaging in menial work or facing the greatest of personal tragedies. Viktor Frankl, the great Austrian psychiatrist, felt that a sense of meaning was the single most critical factor in surviving the unbelievable atrocities of a German concentration camp, including abuse, starvation and even typhus infection.

Today, spirituality is considered an important part of secular life. No longer is it necessary to cloister oneself to invoke the sacred. We are surrounded by a growing chorus of personal-growth groups, books, tapes, men's movements, women's movements, children's movements and so on. Many of these groups are attempting to fill the void that has occurred in the last fifty years since the relative breakup of extended and nuclear families. Basically, society is responding to its existential crisis by seeking meaning.

Even though technology has partially trivialized the transcendent and organized religions have lost members, while society has tumultuously and radically changed, strong spiritual countermovements have arisen and may become proportionately stronger as the machinist evolution nears its end of affluence, if not of influence.

Concomitant with the spiritual decay of the Vietnam War, the redeeming humanistic psychology movement was spawned, followed by the transpersonal psychology movement and then the holistic health and medicine movement. Humanistic psychology has emphasized the importance of the individual, of feeling, of self-actualization or what Carl Jung would have called individuation, that is, the movement of the individual toward ultimate adult maturity. The transpersonal psychology movement emphasizes a connectedness with spirit, soul or God. The holistic health movement emphasizes the importance of the spiritual aspects of life in overall well-being. In general, all of these trends use the concept of body, mind and spirit as being parts of the whole.

THE MEANING OF SPIRITUALITY

Perhaps no word is more complex and potentially misunderstood than the word "spirit" or "spirituality." Charles Fillmore, founder of Unity, in his book *The Twelve Powers of Man* emphasized twelve faculties that he felt represented spirituality: faith, strength, discrimination or judgment, love, power, imagination, understanding, will, order, zeal, renunciation or elimination and life-conserving. Some of those words are very difficult to describe and understand. I explain some below as I understand them.

Faith: He discussed the faith of Abraham, who offered up his son Isaac, the faith of Moses's parents, who hid him for three months when he was born, and the faith by which the walls of Jerico fell.

Strength, stability, or steadfastness: David, trusting in his spiritual strength, overcame the greater size and physical power of Goliath. The strength referred to here is the strength of spirituality, not that of physical power.

Wisdom or judgment: Solomon chose wisdom above riches and honor. Judgment, discrimination, intuition and the mere act of "knowing" are all aspects of wisdom.

Regenerating love: Here the meaning of unconditional love is essential. Love is not liking, it is "the desire to do good to others."

Power, dominion, mastery: Here, again, Fillmore is talking about spiritual power, not physical power.

Imagination, regeneration: Early in this century, the autonomic nervous system was called "the imaginative nervous system" because it was known that imagery affects the function of the body, and through proper imagery, regeneration can occur.

Understanding: Fillmore is referring to spiritual understanding or spiritual illumination.

Love: Ultimately, love is the greatest spiritual attitude. Love means not necessarily liking to nurture or help others without conditions or reward but desiring to do so nevertheless. Unconditional love without judgment, with no need to know why, is often said to be the essence of Christian faith or of God.

Grace: The most intriguing attitude relating to healing is grace. *Webster's* dictionary defines grace as "charm, elegance, attractiveness, especially of a delicate, slender, refined, light or unlabored kind. . . . unconstrained and undeserved divine favor or goodwill, God's loving mercy displayed to man for a salvation of his soul." In religious terms, grace implies complete acceptance and forgiveness by God. Essentially that is another aspect of unconditional love by God. Grace completely defies explanation or reason. It just IS. Beyond spirituality is a belief in Grace.

I have reflected upon the attributes of spirituality for much of my life. I list them here in order of importance, as I see them. I encourage you to adapt this list, to make it your own. Though your list may vary somewhat from mine, upon closer examination, the attitudes on your list may be synonyms of the ones on my list. I believe you must integrate the attitudes into your everyday thoughts and actions so as to retain good health.

Forgiveness: Overall the most important single attitude for healing is forgiveness. Carrying a grudge is like taking poison yourself and expecting it to kill your worst enemy.

Tolerance: Acceptance of human differences, beliefs and behaviors, without being judgmental. Tolerance does not condone harmful actions by or toward other people. The ability to celebrate diversity precludes having truly harmful thoughts and actions.

Serenity: An ability to be at peace, especially when there is turmoil around you.

Love: Unconditional desire to help or aid others.

Compassion: A noncritical attitude, compassion for those who are less fortunate or undergoing personal trauma.

Charity: A desire to share with those less fortunate.

Motivation: An inner drive to accomplish.

Joy: Appreciation and enjoyment in the beauty of life.

Faith: That the purpose of life is good.

Hope: That the future will be better.

Confidence: Belief in self.

Courage: Strength to face obstacles.

Will: Ability to express and pursue one's needs and desires.

Reason: Logic and rationality.

Wisdom: Dispassionate discernment and ability to choose the best solution for all concerned.

SPIRITUAL ATTITUDE INVENTORY

This simple questionnaire can assist you if you want to assess your spiritual attitudes. The questions suggest areas on which to reflect regarding your own personal spiritual strengths or weaknesses.

As you read each of the following items to yourself, get a sense of whether your emotional response is agreement or disagreement. If you feel strong agreement, mark ++. If you get mild agreement, mark +. If you get no response at all, mark it 0. If you feel a mild disagreement, mark –. If you are aware of strong disagreement, mark ––. It sometimes happens that people are in agreement in general (which would be a +) and are simultaneously aware of an uneasy feeling that argues or presents a single exception. In such a case, it is permissible to answer + – to reflect this conflict; this would be preferable to marking 0 if you really are getting a mixed response.

Strong agreement ++

Neutral 0

Mild disagreement –

Mild agreement +

Strong disagreement – –

(Mixed responses are possible.)

_____ I have forgiven everyone who has wronged me.

_____ I forgive those who unintentionally wrong me.

_____ I forgive those who purposefully wrong me.

_____ When I tell those who have wronged me what they have done, I expect them to apologize or repent.

_____ I have sometimes wronged or harmed others.

_____ I apologize when I wrong others.

_____ I expect others to forgive me when I apologize.

_____ I helped someone else within the last week.

_____ I walked and talked with someone I love during the last week.

_____ I participate in a spiritual practice regularly.

_____ I believe that my attitude each day is more important than attending church.

_____ I believe my affliction(s) was given to me by God as part of a divine plan.

_____ I believe God is wrathful and punishes sinners.

_____ I have lots of friends and see/visit them often.

_____ I pray regularly for myself and others.

_____ I believe the most important goal of life is service to God or others.

_____ I prayed for someone else yesterday and today.

_____ I often (more than once a week) watch the sunset or sunrise with a feeling of reverence.

_____ I read religious or inspirational materials at least once a week.

_____ I attend a fun event or listen to good music at least once a week.

_____ I meditate, pray, or think about the beauty of life regularly.

_____ Everyone is born a sinner.

_____ Humankind is basically bad.

_____ I believe hypnosis is the work of the Devil.

_____ I believe everyone has a right to his or her beliefs.

_____ I believe that those who do not share my religious beliefs are sinners and likely to go to Hell.

_____ God does not forgive sinners unless the debts of their sins are paid.

_____ If your beliefs are different from mine, you cannot help me.

_____ My spiritual/religious beliefs are:
a. strong _____
b. correct and right _____

_____ I feel calm and serene most of the time.

_____ When I become frustrated, I pause and calm myself.

_____ I feel compassion for all other human beings.

_____ I go out of my way to help other persons.

_____ I know I can attain my goals.

_____ I believe I can accomplish anything to which I apply myself adequately.

_____ I will apply myself enough to accomplish my goals.

_____ I feel great joy in my life.

_____ I can face whatever life offers.

_____ I believe I can learn from my problems.

_____ I willingly or lovingly contribute to help others less fortunate than I.

_____ I believe tomorrow will be a better day.

_____ I believe in a benevolent God.

_____ I believe in life after death.

_____ I believe I have a soul that survives death.

_____ I believe one dies and goes to Heaven or Hell.

_____ I believe in reincarnation.

_____ Reincarnation is an evil concept.

_____ I have the willpower to accomplish my goals.

_____ I am wise enough to make the right choices.

_____ I make rational, reasonable choices.

_____ I feel love for all other human beings.

_____ I bless all other human beings.

_____ I bless all who have wronged me.

_____ My life is meaningful.

7

Sacred Healing:
Real, Unreal,
or Possible?

To most patients, simple relief of symptoms is adequate proof of cure. Unfortunately, for many illnesses cure is more difficult to prove scientifically. Although my goal for this book is to show unequivocal proof of sacred healing, an understanding of the foundation for scientific proof is crucial so as to grasp the remarkable nature of a Sacred Healer.

From a physician's point of view, very few illnesses have enough scientific documentation to prove that they are physical illnesses. That is, a fractured bone is clearly a physical illness. It usually takes six to twelve weeks for healing of a fracture. If a sacred healer could lay on hands and cause the bone to heal within two weeks, that would "prove" effectiveness. In type I or childhood diabetes, that is, diabetes that begins before age thirty-five, it is generally believed in medicine that this is not reversible and the patient will require insulin throughout life. When the onset of diabetes occurs after age thirty-five, it is often controllable by diet, physical exercise, and even deep relaxation training. (Most physicians still do not offer these alternatives and just put the patient on drugs and may suggest dietary control.) It would be difficult for sacred healing to "prove" cure of a type II adult onset diabetic, whereas reversal of type I would be dramatic. Cancer is perhaps the most dramatic illness. "Spontaneous" healing of cancer is indeed a very rare event. Thus cancer above all other illness offers the best opportunity for *proof* of healing.

CONVENTIONAL MEDICINE'S VIEWPOINT

What is real or genuine? Hypertension or high blood pressure is perhaps a prime example of the dilemma in medicine. Most physicians would admit that hypertension is to some extent the result of stress, and yet stress reduction is rarely recommended adequately or taught. For many years it was believed that sodium was the major culprit in hypertension. There is now some evidence that chloride may be more important than sodium. It is also now known that almost all hypertensive patients are deficient in calcium and even more deficient in magnesium. But these replacements are rarely recommended by physicians. Instead, they prescribe drugs that usually (after a trial of several different drugs) will bring the blood pressure under control. Such drugs often cause complications, however, even stroke, and frequently loss of sexual potency in men. Drugs offer at best something of a standoff—they can control the blood pressure but at a significant psychological and physiological cost.

Dr. Elmer Green at the Menninger Foundation, who introduced temperature biofeedback for control of migraine headaches more than twenty-five years ago, at least twenty years ago demonstrated that 80 percent of hypertensive patients could bring their blood pressure under control with temperature biofeedback. His results have been sustained for almost two decades, and yet the medical profession rejects this, and physicians often consider biofeedback itself to be only "placebo." Eighty percent success is hardly placebo, and the control of hypertension with biofeedback is genuine, but because it has not had the kind of financial backing that supports a new drug, it has not been accepted by the medical profession. Such are the philosophical dilemmas in medicine today.

In the medicinal community, there is virtually never total agreement on either diagnosis or therapy, even when a school of thought is shared. The conflict between allopathy (the conventional practice of M.D.s) and holistic medicine is even greater.

For example, Andrew Taylor Still, an M.D., introduced osteopathy in the late nineteenth century. He attempted to have it accepted at the University of Kansas, which had been founded by family members. But his concept that abnormal position, particularly of the vertebrae, produced pressure on arteries and resulted in dysfunction that could be corrected by manipulation was soundly rejected by the medical profession. Osteopaths were treated almost as contemptuously as were chiropractors by allopaths until the mid-1960s, when the AMA suddenly agreed to accept osteopaths as being equally trained and offered osteopaths the opportunity to drop their D.O.s and become M.D.s just with the stroke of a pen. Some 2,000 did so, but most retained their osteopathic roots.

Homeopathy is even more controversial than osteopathy. Samuel Hahnemann (1755–1843), a German physician, introduced homeopathy at a time of "uncertainty, contention, and contradiction" as one German medical professor called his age. Hahnemann was quite disillusioned with many of the medical practices of his day, which included leeching, bloodletting and purging. He introduced substances to healthy individuals and made a detailed record of the symptoms they produced. He then diluted those substances many thousands or millions of times to treat patients whose symptoms were identical with the symptom pattern developed when that substance was administered in larger doses. Hahnemann called this the law of similars, that is, *like cures like.* In allopathic practice, drugs are used to control or suppress the symptoms of an illness. In homeopathy, extremely dilute amounts of substances that "cause" the symptoms are given to desensitize or strengthen the body's inherent healing ability. Allopathy supports the law of opposites; homeopathy promotes the law of similars.

Allopathy has dominated scientific medicine for at least seventy-five years, with emphasis largely being placed on drugs and surgery as remedies. Almost all therapy outside those remedies has been rejected, suppressed, criticized or attacked verbally and legally. Thus, the oldest forms of healing—acupuncture, nutrition, sacred healing, herbs, massage, manipulation and psychotherapy (for the most part)—have been largely rejected.

THE PLACEBO EFFECT

Logical, systematic, and mathematical principles are the basis of conventional medicine. Proof of efficacy and safety are accomplished by double-blind, crossover research studies. Double-blind means that neither the patient nor the therapist knows what the patient is receiving. Generally, one-third to one-half of the patients are given a "sugar pill" or placebo, and the other half or two-thirds are given what is thought to be the "active" drug. The purpose of this approach is to prove that a given treatment is statistically more likely to improve a specific symptom or physical condition to a greater degree than a placebo would accomplish under the same circumstances.

In cross-over studies, after an initial treatment period ranging from one week to a month or more, the subjects who received placebo receive the "real" drug, and those who received the drug now receive the placebo. Again, neither the physician or nurse dispensing the medication nor the patient knows whether the patient is receiving placebo or an "active" drug. Theoretically, this allows any differences between the two to become more apparent, but often the differences still remain small.

Statistics are wonderful. A difference of only one or two percent can "prove" that the treatment is superior to placebo. But is that really superior? Often I personally would prefer to use the placebo!

Double-blind studies are tedious and difficult to conduct. One needs to look at many different factors, not just a single symptom. Results are subject to hundreds or thousands of variables. For instance, in looking at hypertension, smoking, caffeine intake, sugar intake, calcium, magnesium, body weight, genetics and physical exercise are all variables that can influence blood pressure significantly. In fact, these same variables are virtually equally important in affecting diabetes. And there is, of course, individual biochemical variability. Some individuals metabolize carbohydrates easily; others have trouble with many carbohydrates, not just simple sugars but even starches. "Jack Sprat could eat no fat; his wife could eat no lean" is indeed a very real aspect of life. Blood cholesterol and triglycerides are also affected by many different factors, including sugar intake, caffeine, nicotine, alcohol, exercise, weight and genetics.

Efficacy for almost any drug undergoing reasonably vigorous investigation is established by proof that the drug is more effective than a placebo (frequently a sugar pill or an injection of distilled, sterile water). And as indicated earlier, the drug needs to show an efficacy of only a few percent above that of placebo to be considered "effective." Placebos typically average 35 percent effectiveness. Drugs must succeed by only 2 percent to be considered therapeutic if the 2 percent superiority is consistent in a few thousand patients.

Such were the findings of Dr. Herb Benson, the Harvard internist who demonstrated in 1979, through rigid scientific study, that no treatment of angina pectoris, either by drugs or surgery, was better than the 35 percent placebo effect.[1] But physicians who believed in their treatment reported an astounding 90 percent success rate. (The remaining 10 percent of people failed to respond, which is true in the best of cases.) Absolutely no pill or surgery safely achieves that success, including coronary bypass surgery and all the drugs used for angina. The physician's belief—and indeed the patient's belief or intent—is the final factor in determining healing.

Personally, I prefer results that show a drug is at least 75 percent effective. This is more than twice the average placebo and is rarely achieved by any drug.

U.S. medicine has emphasized X-ray, blood chemistry and electrocardiograms. Neurologists and neurosurgeons have often relied on electroencephalograms (EEG). Interestingly, now that we have computerized analysis of EEGs, we find many more variabilities than were apparent even to a trained encephalographer. Computers can now measure differences of less than 1 percent between the two sides of the brain. These can be documented both in percentages and in graphic pictures. Increasingly, such "brain maps" are becoming accepted by the medical profession, especially among those who are experienced and well read in this subject. Blood tests, which are relatively stable, are also another good test of therapeutic effectiveness. DHEA or dehydroepiandrosterone, in my opinion the single most important hormone in the human body, is reported in the literature to be very stable, changing not more than 15 percent at various times of day or with different seasons. Thus a change of 25 percent, 50 percent or 100 percent in DHEA is scientifically remarkable.

THE DANGER OF DRUGS

Drugs can produce a remarkable variety and range of side effects or even serious complications. For every drug included in the *Physicians' Desk Reference*, the list of complications, adverse effects and warnings is enough to scare most patients. These so-called side effects can be somewhat minor problems or major illnesses. That is, drugs may cause both a lack of well-being as well as illness.

Although the dictionary defines disease and illness as being similar, some writers like me prefer to use the word dis-ease to indicate symptoms without a major ailment. Dizziness, agitation, insomnia, drowsiness, constipation and diarrhea are among the most common possible symptoms. They may occur spontaneously with no clear-cut "cause" and may occur with placebo as well as with drugs.

With most drugs, these particular symptoms are only slightly more common than they are with placebo. On the other hand, most mood-altering drugs, such as antidepressants and tranquilizers, and most cardiovascular drugs (those used for hypertension or other heart disorders) have a much higher incidence of these common symptoms as well as more serious ones. The major reason that dizziness, agitation, insomnia and so forth are so common is that those are symptoms associated with stress. Mental and emotional anxiety can easily produce those particular symptoms. Mood and cardiovascular drugs work to alter the stress response; thus they may add significantly to the natural background stress level. In general, these relatively common symptomatic side effects are not serious or life threatening.

But because there are safer, less disruptive alternatives, why use drugs as a first course of therapeutic action? And because placebo works as well as many drugs, we should rethink the drug habit that is pervasive in our medical establishment.

ALLOPATHIC VS. HOLISTIC MEDICINE

The crowning achievement of allopathic scientific medicine is the ability of M.D.s to make a specific diagnosis. Congestive heart failure, diabetes, hypertension, various forms of cancer and so forth are easily diagnosed. Although remarkable advances in surgery have been made, such procedures would be unusable without proper diagnoses. Truly miraculous diagnostic tools are available today, such as MRI (magnetic resonance imaging), enabling detailed evaluation of the brain, spinal cord and many other organs with a clarity often beyond that which is visible even surgically. Allopathic diagnostic capability is truly superb.

Once a diagnosis is made, and even with advanced drugs and surgical therapy, just how good is modern medicine compared with holistic medicine? We probably will never know the answer to this question. It is the belief of most holistic and alternative physicians that modern medicine is particularly good in treating acute illness and particularly inept at treating chronic illness. Acute illnesses include significant illnesses and injuries, serious infections, fractures and shock from a radical, serious drop in blood pressure (if it occurs in a hospital). Chronic illnesses include cancer, rheumatoid arthritis, lupus erythematosus, osteoarthritis, multiple sclerosis, diabetes, emphysema, asthma, congestive heart failure, chronic pain, migraine and stroke.

Though symptom control clearly can often improve one's quality of life, that is the only remedy conventional medicine offers for most other illnesses, not "cure." Regardless of advanced cancer treatments, 50 percent of patients still die within five years from many types of cancer. Also, cancer chemotherapy can destroy or radically alter the quality of a patient's life. Thus, if surgery or antibiotics cannot cure the problem, safe alternatives should be used if they either cure or improve quality of life.

A few of the diseases for which medicine is only partially helpful I refer to as semi-orphan diseases. Although some physicians would argue with my list, I challenge them to "cure" most of these illnesses. Indeed, even the quality of life is often minimally affected by drugs or surgery. Semi-orphan diseases are many types of cancer, rheumatoid arthritis, lupus erythematosus, multiple sclerosis, chronic hepatitis, stroke, retinitis pigmentosa, macular degeneration, allergies, chronic fatigue syndrome and depression.

STRESS AND HEALTH

Stress is the common denominator in all dis-ease as well as in serious illnesses. Those physicians who have emphasized holistic and alternative approaches understand the stress reaction well.

Hans Selye (1907–1982), the brilliant physician who introduced us to the concept of stress, discovered the correlation between one's state of health and stress well over sixty years ago. Thousands of scientific papers have documented the multifaceted face of stress. Essentially, when there is enough pressure—physical, chemical, emotional or electromagnetic—to cause a doubling in the amount of adrenaline in the blood, then blood sugar goes up, increased insulin is produced, and a stress response occurs. Selye called this "an alarm reaction."

If one is exposed to the same stressor repeatedly, after a short period of time the stress reaction does not occur. This is the stage of *adaptation*. Selye emphasized, however, that every time one adapts to a stress, the threshold for new stress is lowered.

Even sub-threshold amounts of stress are cumulative. For instance, it takes one cigarette to raise adrenaline production to roughly twice the normal level. A third of a cigarette has very little effect. It takes a cup of coffee to pro-duce an alarm reaction. But one third of a cup of coffee, a third of a cigarette and two teaspoons of sugar will add together to produce an alarm reaction. Eventually, individuals begin to "burn out." This is the stage of *maladaptation* which, according to Selye, is the common feature of all significant ill-nesses. And eventually, when the body cannot cope at all, a terminal state occurs, which Selye called "exhaustion."

To a large extent, modern medicine minimizes the role of stress, even though for more than twenty-five years numerous reports have demonstrated the diagnostic and therapeutic importance of stress management.

Many of the reports related to stress are as extraordinary as a magnetic resonance image (or MRI), one of our prime allopathic diagnostic tools. For an in–depth understanding of stress, read *Mind as Healer, Mind as Slayer*, by Kenneth Pelletier; *Beyond Biofeedback*, by Elmer and Alyce Green; *90 Days to Self-Health*, by C. Norman Shealy; and *Who Gets Sick?*, by Blair Justice.

IS SPIRITUAL BELIEF A PLACEBO?

The placebo effect is surely some component of sacred heal-ing as well as of *all* healing. Actually, in the most rigidly scientific studies, placebo therapy is usually 35 percent effective. Thus medical effectiveness is measured as being greater than placebo—though often only a few percent above placebo, or "barely above the positive" as Ingelfinger stated.

Early in the 1900s, Emil Coue, the French pharmacist, was cited by European physicians as having cured tens of thousands of patients. He accomplished this through a simple positive affirmation, "Every day in every way I am getting better and better." Although Coue's work is generally dismissed as a placebo at best, a placebo's power may be stronger than any drug or surgery because it represents an individual's belief. Mocked by the American Medical Association, Coue may still have the last laugh.

During the last two decades, psychoneuroimmunology has become a major new science. It is now known that the immune system is more powerfully influenced by attitude and belief than virtually all other normal factors combined. Norman Cousins awakened us to the healing power of one of the great spiritual fruits—laughter. He initially wrote an article in *The New England Journal of Medicine* entitled, "Anatomy of an Illness."[2] It is one of the few articles written by a layman ever published in our most prestigious medical journal. Later *Anatomy of an Illness* became a best-selling book. Essentially, Cousins reported that laughter and intravenous vitamin C brought under control a serious and temporarily invaliding illness, probably rheumatoid spondylitis.

While a patient's belief is a key factor in his or her healing, sacred healing can also take place without the patient's knowledge or participation. Absent healing is as enigmatic as grace to healing. The healing occurs without an individual knowing of an interdiction by way of prayer or a sacred healer. Convincing evidence of the efficacy of absent healing by prayer has been demonstrated in a study of patients in the cardiac care unit. In a double-blind study, without the patients' knowledge, half of a group of patients had absent prayer directed toward them while the other half did not. Those who received absent prayer had a statistically significantly greater survival rate and a shorter hospital stay. Those persons for whom there was no specific group prayer did not do as well.[3] These results might have been even more striking if we knew whether those who did not receive the group prayer had families praying for them or were intervening in their own way with prayer. In other words, some of the controls may have done better because of unreported prayer assistance.

Edgar Cayce, one of the most quoted intuitives of all time, often stated that physical illnesses were the result of unsatisfactory attitudes. "No one can hate his neighbor and not have stomach or liver trouble. No one can be jealous and allow the anger of same and not have upset digestion or heart disorder" (Reading 4021-1). Or, "Hate, malice, and jealousy only create poisons within the minds, souls, and bodies of people" (Reading 3312-1). He emphasized always that one should reach for or emphasize the ideal. The fruits of the spirit—love, kindness and patience—were repeatedly pointed to as essential spiritual ideals. Though essentially a spiritual diagnostician and not a spiritual healer, Cayce has benefited hundreds of thousands of people. Through his Search for God Program, he referred to the essentials of spirituality more often than perhaps any other concept in his almost 15,000 intuitive readings.

TESTIMONIES OF SACRED HEALING

As Dr. Nolen emphasized in his book, healers have a 70 percent success rate, but he thought most of their success was due to placebo in psychosomatic illnesses. Although I will report specific medical records in detail in a later chapter, I think it is valuable to read some of the anecdotal evidence of sacred healing. Physicians might dismiss the cures cited in this section even though a number of the letters were sent by physicians or licensed healthcare professionals. You can dismiss one white crow, but can you dismiss a whole flock?

Situation 1

A woman writes, "I have been suffering from rheumatoid arthritis for the past ten years; fortunately, since you began your treatments, the pain and symptoms of the arthritis have gone into remission—I am able to work out and enjoy swimming, something which was not even possible to think about during the past painful ten years. I am very happy and energetic now, like never before."

Situation 2

An M.D. ophthalmologist writes in January 1996, "Mr. _____ has been my patient since 1986 and was under my supervision. His vision gradually was lost due to macular degeneration in both eyes so that he was not able to drive. At present his vision is improved after visiting Mr. Parvarandeh, and he is able to drive because of improving vision in both eyes."

Situation 3

A chiropractor writes that her chronically ill mother "came

out of her silence immediately. Her overall manner was changed. She started smiling and talking, and suddenly I felt there was actually somebody present next to me. The lacrimation of her eyes and nose stopped, which was very plentiful due to complete bilateral obstruction of her lacrimal ducts. Her leg pain was improved. My husband excitedly greeted me saying he noticed complete change in my mother's behavior."

Situation 4

A psychologist and director of a major pain clinic wrote in March 1996, "I have been quite amazed by the progress shown by several of my patients who have seen you."

Situation 5

A New York M.D. wrote in March 1996, "I was profoundly impressed with your capability to provide significant and documented—need I say almost miraculous—benefit to a large variety of often very difficult cases in the face of prior unsuccessful attempts by the best Western medicine has to offer."

Situation 6

A Philadelphia scientist wrote in March 1996, "We were amazed at your extraordinary capacity to diagnose rapidly and treat patients with subtle energy and the power of intention in our presence, some of whom have lasting pain relief or other improved condition as a direct result of your treatment. Everyone I spoke with following your visit here is greatly impressed with your abilities."

Situation 7

In May 1996 two parents wrote, "Our son was born on 4/4/93. After three fractures in his first fifteen months of life, a diagnosis of osteogenesis imperfecta was made. Our son had a broken bone every three months or so, until October 1995 when we were able to meet you (Ostad Parvarandeh). After five treatments our son is fine now. He fell several times. He runs. He plays with other children, and we enjoy watching him play and run."

Situation 8

A board-certified M.D. family physician wrote in June 1996, "I have witnessed the healing of illnesses that go far beyond the capability of conventional Western medicine."

Situation 9

A patient diagnosed at Mayo Clinic with Kugelberg-Weilander, a rare, progressive degenerative disorder, was reported by a professor of anesthesiology to have improvement, "including an increase in strength and a feeling of being energized."

Situation 10

A doctor of oriental medicine wrote in July 1996 that his son had had serious problems with Crohn's disease for five years, with frequent diarrhea; he had lost forty pounds. Initially Ostad treated the son over the phone for five minutes. Immediately the diarrhea ceased and the pain was less severe. After a second and final treatment, "symptoms dramatically decreased. He began tolerating normal foods, and over the next four months totally stopped taking all medications and gained thirty-eight pounds."

Situation 11

An M.D. and an independent physical therapist both wrote in July 1996 that a patient with lupus erythematosus and myasthenia gravis reported, after treatments by Master Parvarandeh, "a noticeable increase in energy and well-being and feels this has allowed her to progress with her strengthening."

Situation 12

A father wrote in August 1996 that his daughter, stunted

by severe psoriasis, grew one inch in four weeks under treatment by Ostad.

Situation 13

A man with severe post-traumatic glaucoma with multiple unsuccessful surgeries reported, "After a few sessions with Ostad Parvarandeh, my pain and the condition of the eye was much improved, to the point that there are no more medications or surgeries needed."

Situation 14

A father wrote that his son had battled for two years with a deep cough so severe that it interrupted his sleep frequently. Numerous physicians and specialists were unable to help. After only three healing sessions with Ostad, "his symptoms have completely disappeared."

Situation 15

A doctor of oriental medicine and acupuncture wrote that he had observed Ostad "greatly improve and cure the ailments of different patients such as cancer, incurable viruses, seizures and even blindness, and the Master has not only cured the patients, but has also rejuvenated the life back into their spirits." He said that even manic depression and schizophrenia have been no challenge for Master Parvarandeh.

Situation 16

A New Jersey physician wrote, "I witnessed the effect of his healing power on several patients." He then goes on to describe eight patients:

1. The first patient was a fifty-eight-year-old doctor who underwent spinal fusion surgery in 1987 and developed paralysis of the right lower limb due to complication of surgery, later confirmed by MRI examinations. The surgeons were not interested in further surgery. After his first thera-peutic session with Ostad, a very fine movement was noted in his right toes. After forty sessions of therapy, the patient, who had been paralyzed, could walk with a walker and crutches, and is currently practicing medicine in his office. I'm not aware of any nonsurgical intervention or therapy that could ameliorate such organic spinal cord injuries in such a short period of time.

2. A thirty-two-year-old woman, the wife of a doctor, developed amenorrhea and galactorrhea, which persisted four years after giving birth to her second child. The patient was treated by Mr. Parvarandeh for three sessions. Her symptoms disappeared and her menstrual cycles were normal. In the first

session the patient was seen in person by Mr. Parvarandeh, and the next two sessions were done over the phone.

3. A thirty-five-year-old woman, the wife of a doctor, developed a severe frontal throbbing headache. In spite of all physical examinations and laboratory and paraclinical tests such as MRI and CT scans, no definite cause was identified. Ophthalmologic exams were normal. It was diagnosed as a nervous headache, and she used pain killers. Mr. Parvarandeh diagnosed the headache as being due to minimal liver dysfunction. It is noteworthy that all liver function tests were within the normal range. After a few sessions of therapy in which Mr. Parvarandeh was concentrating on the liver, her headache disappeared. This is a new idea not known by medical doctors that liver dysfunction, even in the presence of normal function tests, could exist and lead to headache; it is believed there is no known medication for such treatment.

4. After transfer of energy to the liver of several patients with hypercholesterolemia and hypertriglyceridemia by Mr. Parvarandeh, the blood levels of triglycerides and cholesterol dropped significantly. There was no medication that could do the same.

5. A sixty-seven-year-old surgeon who has liver cirrhosis developed thrombocytopenia. After receiving the healing

energy of Mr. Parvarandeh, platelets increased from 20,000 to 50,000 and the size of the spleen decreased.

6. I have also witnessed the decrease of chest pain in patients with proven angina pectoris and myocardial infarction.

7. A patient with frozen shoulder, after fracture of the head of the humerus, regained full function of the shoulder joint after a few sessions of therapy by Mr. Parvarandeh.

8. A five-year-old girl was diagnosed with alveolar soft part sarcoma of the right leg in 1986. The tumor showed histological evidence of muscular and vascular invasion. Pathologic diagnosis was confirmed at a center in England and the United States. The patient was referred to a center in England where she received a course of chemotherapy, and she was discharged with a diagnosis of metastatic sarcoma to the lung with no further therapy. She has since then been under treatment by healing power of Mr. Parvarandeh and is still alive and doing well ten years after the initial diagnosis. This case is one of the very rare long-term survivals of metastatic sarcoma, and may be the only case of long-term survival in metastatic sarcoma to the lung.

Although all of these sound like anecdotes, I have medical documentation of all but one of them. These cases are only a small sample of apparent, miraculous sacred healing power. In none of these cases does conventional medicine have anything to offer. Of course, it is also worth noting that Ostad's treatments are free. He does not charge for his services. Most sacred healers have no set fee and either accept a "love offering" or refuse any payment. This sacred healing includes faith and, at least occasionally, Grace.

8

The Brain,
the Mind, and
the Spirit

Although we understand much of the anatomy and physiology (electricity and chemistry) of the brain, we understand much less about the mind and, scientifically, nothing about the spirit. We can measure physical, chemical and electrical energy. The energy we call spiritual cannot be measured with test tubes, X-rays or oscilloscopes. I'll talk more later about what we understand of electromagnetic energy. Now let us examine the energetics of brain, mind and behavior, especially in relation to spiritual beliefs and attitudes.

THE CONNECTION BETWEEN
THE BRAIN AND THE MIND

An observable but poorly measurable energetic component of sacred healing is the relationship between the brain and mind. Though the brain has been studied extensively—it already has been examined more intimately than any other human organ—there is still much to do. And, while we know a lot about the brain, some of its aspects remain mysterious. For instance, what is consciousness? What do we mean by *conscious, unconscious,* and *superconscious?* We use these terms without tangible, measurable proof of their meaning.

Questions involving the brain-mind relationship remain unanswered despite thousands of years of philosophical and theological inquiry. We still don't know what constitutes the mind. How does the mind interface or interact with the brain? What is the relation of one human brain/mind with other human minds? How does the "living" aspect of plants or animals relate to the human mind? Is a human soul involved with the mind? (Remember, 90 percent of humanity believes the soul survives physical death.) Sometimes common sense is more fruitful and enlightening in dealing with mysteries and ambiguities. For instance, artists, poets, novelists, cartoonists and satirists all make a living interpreting various aspects of mind and behavior.

Much evidence concerning the effects of attitudes, beliefs and emotions—all attributes of personality—has been evaluated and measured. The pursuits of the scholarly fields of philosophy, theology, psychology and psychiatry are concerned with study of attitudes, beliefs, emotions, personality and behavior.

These definitions come from the *Random House College Dictionary* (New York, 1984).

Attitudes: Manner, disposition, feeling, position toward a person or thing.

Beliefs: Something believed; an opinion or conviction. Confidence in the truth or existence of something not immediately susceptible to rigorous proof. Confidence, faith or trust.

Emotions: An affective state of consciousness in which joy, sorrow, fear, hate or the like is experienced as distinguished from cognitive and volitional states of consciousness: usually accompanied by certain physiological changes, as increased heartbeat, respiration or the like, and often overt manifestation, as crying, shaking or laughing. An instance of this, as love, hate, sorrow or fear.

Despite universal spiritual unifying principles, uncivilized societies and brutal individual human behavior continue to exist today. These actions are far more cruel and senseless than any aspect of animal behavior. We see instances of this "inhumanity" throughout the world, in Ireland, the Middle East, in the former Soviet Union and in Bosnia. In the United States, crime abounds—rape, murder, robbery, extortion, embezzlement and drug abuse—indications of flagrant, serious disregard for life and well-being.

Most civilized societies uphold a single, great universal commandment, often called The Golden Rule. Fortunately, most people practice what it preaches. The great world religions all observe this rule. Its underlying meaning, which is to treat other people well or they will get even with you, is clear to any seven-year-old child. Even if one intrinsically has no compassion or desire to help others, the Rule denotes a commonsense mode of conduct. To most of us, it appears logical that we should not purposefully harm someone else. The remaining minority of humanity with truly criminal minds and personalities make life more unpleasant for the majority!

THE HEALTH CONSEQUENCES OF EMOTIONS, ATTITUDES AND BEHAVIORS

At some level we all suffer the consequences of negative emotions and behavior. All illness and ultimately death result from cumulative total stress: physical, chemical, emotional, mental, electromagnetic and spiritual. Spiritual distress results, in part, from disregarding The Golden Rule. Perhaps the most important human lesson is to learn to live that rule consciously, subconsciously, unconsciously and superconsciously, individually and collectively, at all levels of our being.

In the name of world religions, despite their professed belief in the Rule, people have been exterminated and mutilated down through history. How can religious leaders justify such extreme harm to others? What is the impact of such inhumane behavior on the physiological, electromagnetic and chemical balances of those cruel leaders and of their underlings who carry out such insane orders?

Why have churches sown so much guilt? Maybe they cannot control their members except by insisting on extensive dogma other than The Golden Rule. What are the subtle effects of religious "prohibition" of masturbation, sex outside of marriage, homosexual acts and contraception? With the exception of marital infidelity, none of these acts harms another human being. Not only has there been little scientific study of the philosophical questions mentioned here, it may not be possible to study them effectively. However, it is obvious to those of us who study human behavior that these broader philosophical social issues must be as pervasively harmful as air, water, soil and electromagnetic pollution. Environmentalists emphasize the negative health effects of pollution. I would equally emphasize the negative health effects of hypocritical inhibition of normal and nonharmful behaviors.

Growing evidence indicates media violence increases violence among children and adults. Thus in the "collective unconscious" the overall energetic field contains negative influences that theoretically may adversely affect all of us, some more than others.

Mahatma Gandhi popularized an awareness of seven types of social sins:

- Politics without *principles*
- Wealth without *work*
- Pleasure without *conscience*
- Knowledge without *character*
- Science without *humanity*
- Commerce without *morality*
- Worship without *sacrifice*

I would add an eighth: intolerance of normal, healthy, nonharmful behavior! In Springfield, Missouri, where the Shealy Institute is located, "tolerance" was removed as a community value because some religious fundamentalists refused to be tolerant. When part of society forces its interpretation of right and wrong on all others, we approach totalitarianism.

Beyond individual responsibility is the responsibility of groups, corporations and government. Why do so many corporations rape the earth and/or lie in ways that ultimately rob millions of people of security, health or even life? Nuclear and chemical contamination are threats to the earth. And few are willing to evaluate or consider the health effects of unprecedented electromagnetic pollution. How can tobacco companies continue to be accomplices to virtual mass murder? How can food companies distort the quality of their foods? How can pesticides and herbicides banned in the United States be exported to Third World countries, poisoning farmers and their families there as well as those of us here who buy imported foods? What about soil and water erosion and pollution? Ultimately the "sins" will be visited upon future generations.

The reasons for such psychosocial disregard for the common good are not clear. It is also unclear why so many people choose habits and lifestyles that create imbalance, disharmony and dis-ease.

At the individual level, evidence of the adverse effects of

negative thinking and feeling are convincing to anyone willing to examine the facts. Fear, anxiety, guilt, anger and
depression are the major negative emotions. Each of them
evokes a stress reaction, more difficult to evaluate than the
effects of nicotine, caffeine or alcohol, and ultimately more
insidiously pervasive. These gross emotional reactions are
easier to study than the effects of prejudices such as racial or
gender discrimination. What are the individual and collective effects of bigotry? What are the physiological effects in
a person who is subjected to bigotry? When people such as
Mahatma Gandhi or Martin Luther King are struggling for
improvement of human behavior, for righting wrongs, is
their physiology compensated positively? What are the
effects of constant exposure to the suffering of others? Is
there a negative drain from being exposed to the anger or
depression of others? Does a saintly person such as Mother
Theresa receive physiological benefits as well as spiritual
ones from her work with suffering?

Again, these broader questions largely defy scientific
study. But the implications are there from our knowledge of
the effects of anger and depression. Chronic anger is clearly
associated with high blood pressure, migraine and heart
attacks. Chronic depression is clearly associated medically
with cancer. The work of Hans Selye, Kenneth Pelletier,

Hans Eysenck and excellent summaries by Blair Justice provide adequate descriptions of the disease implications of human emotions and behavior. The bottom line is *you cannot afford the luxury of fear, anxiety, anger, guilt or depression*, no matter what the "cause"! And you can't afford prejudice, dislike, hatred, resentment, greed or ignorance (the failure to accept truth or facts). At some level there has to be a physiological negative effect.

Novelists often succeed in portraying an archetypal overview of life. For instance, Robertson Davies captured the essence of the physiologic harm that negative emotions and behavior cause in his outstanding novel, *The Cunning Man*. He shows the impact of psychopathology better than most clinicians or scientists can. Anyone reading his book will be able to understand the end result of a life that has been unfulfilled or damaged by poor self-esteem or extreme bigotry. Unanswered by Davies are questions about lesser emotional dis-stress, petty jealousy, guilt and so on.

Fear, anger, guilt, anxiety, depression, pessimism, prejudice, hatred, resentment and greed sap or zap our health. What are the antidotes? Joy, laughter, happiness, serenity, peacefulness, optimism, forgiveness, patience, tolerance, compassion and love—a desire to do good and help others. These attributes of the spirit enhance health and well-being.

They build beta endorphins, the feel-good, natural narcotics, DHEA and immune competency. Theoretically, if one could exclusively cultivate and maintain these positive attitudes, emotions and behaviors, there might be no need even for sacred healing. Poets, artists, musicians, novelists and some theologians extol the spiritual virtues enumerated above. These fruits of the spirit are worthy of emulation.

The ultimate regulator of brain and mind and, thus, the electromagnetic framework of life is the human spirit. The key to good health is attitude, that is, one's belief in the ultimate goodness of the universe. Relaxation, visualization and meditation are tools for developing spiritual values. Books that promote or discuss a positive approach to life are included in the references at the end of this book.

9

Energy and Electromagnetism

Since the discovery of electricity, electromagnetism has been seen to be the foundation for life energy itself. Although metaphysically oriented individuals describe a fourth dimensional energetic system, currently there is no measurable fourth dimensional alternative energy system. Someday this fourth dimensional energy, often referred to as love, will be harnessed, but at least at present spirit and divine cannot be measured.

DISCOVERY OF ELECTRICITY'S ROLE

In 1600, William Gilbert in his book *DeMagnete* first introduced the concept of electricity and magnetism. He established the difference between electricity (he originated the word) and magnetism, and introduced the concept of magnetic fields. Throughout the seventeenth century, however, such scientists as Descartes and William Harvey believed an "animating force" or "vital spirit" was necessary to the mechanical physics of the body.

Von Guericke invented the first device for generating electricity in 1660. Newton theorized that Descartes's vital principle, or animating force, was an "all pervading ether" that not only filled the universe but also flowed through nerves in the human body to produce the functions we call life.

Early in the eighteenth century, physicist Stephen Gray discovered that some materials were conductors of electricity. We know today that copper is an excellent conductor, whereas wood or glass shield or prevent conduction. Shortly thereafter, Stephen Hales theorized that nerves might function by conducting electrical powers. However, proof of electrical transmission within the body was not conclusive until 1786, when physiologist Luigi Galvani and his associates discovered static electricity could travel from outside the body through a nerve inside the body to make a muscle contract. Thus, Galvani decided that "animal electricity" was the long theorized "vital force."

By the mid-1700s, electricity was being artificially

generated, stored and transmitted. Quickly, this new discovery became a treatment for a variety of illnesses. The first book concerning the topic was *Electrical Medicine*, published in 1752 by Joharen Schaeffer. A nephew of Galvani, Giovanni Aldini, reported significant improvement and even complete rehabilitation of a schizophrenic with transcranial electrical stimulation.

In 1820, Hans Christian Oersted discovered electromagnetism by demonstrating the effect of electricity upon a compass. In the 1830s, Carlo Matteucci first showed that injured tissues generate an electrical current. Pursuing Matteucci's work, DuBois Reymond demonstrated the nerve impulse, the essential mechanism for transfer of information within the nervous system. His colleagues even measured the velocity of a nerve impulse at thirty meters per second.

Julius Bernstein, in 1868, introduced the concept of bioelectricity, created by transfer of ions across cell membranes. Today we know that intracellular potassium and magnesium are higher than extracellular levels, while extracellular sodium and calcium are higher than intracellular bioelectricity. All these ions carry a positive electrical charge. Their movement, positive across a membrane, generates electricity.

With Bernstein's discovery, the machinists of science quickly rejected electricity in favor of the chemical/physics concept, ignoring the fact that the chemical reaction generated electricity! Chemistry was, at that time, easier to measure than subtle electrical energy.

But clinicians are more pragmatic, and thousands of nineteenth-century physicians chose to use electricity to treat a variety of problems. After the 1910 publication of the Flexner Report, science and ultimately the medical community rejected electrotherapy in favor of physics and chemistry. Flexner was hired by the American Medical Association to assess medicine in the United States and to assist the AMA in creating an allopathic monopoly.

Though nonscientific abuses undoubtedly existed in the system, Flexner was a machinist supreme and recommended excommunication of every naturalist concept of health. Osteopathy, acupuncture and homeopathy were targeted in his zest to expunge ineffective concepts. Unfortunately, Flexner's report "threw out the baby with the bath water"; it was accepted as if law.

More than half of all U.S. medical schools and hospitals did not survive Flexner's attack. Homeopathy and acupuncture have marginally existed. Osteopathy barely survived the censorship until the mid-1960s. Perhaps the battle against chiropractics was so strong that the American Medical Association grudgingly accepted osteopathy.

Since 1910 and the Flexner Report, most aspects of life have improved by way of advances in electric technology and electrification of the world. Few of us would opt to give up electric lighting, cooking appliances, radio, TV, computers and so on. Sadly though, the study of two important aspects affecting our health have virtually stopped, that is, the benefits of electrotherapy and the potential negative effects of artificially generated electromagnetism in our environment.

The medical-scientific black hole created by the Flexner Report resulted in the oversight of significant findings in Thomas Edison's lab. He showed the induction of a subjective sensation of flickering light when human volunteers were placed in an alternating on/off magnetic field. That is, a magnetic field turned on and off obviously activated the optic visual system to produce a flicker. Somehow this has to be electricity *induced* in a human by magnetism. The total denial of any impact of electromagnetic fields on life is particularly hard to reconcile with common sense and logic.

Once chemistry became the accepted lifeline of the cell, biochemistry and chemical drugs became the only foundation of modern medicine. In fact, numerous other important electromagnetic experiments were ignored.

- In 1902, a French physician named Leduc reported narcotizing animals with 35 volts of alternating current at 110 cycles per second (Hertz or Hz). Carlotti in 1938 introduced electroshock therapy for schizophrenia and later depression.

- In 1929, Hans Berger discovered the electroencephalogram, electrical rhythm of the brain. Berger postulated a "bioelectric field." Discovered in 1929, the electrocardiogram (EKG or ECG) has been invaluable in the diagnosis of cardiac disease. Later, the electromyogram (EMG) and nerve conduction testing became essential diagnostic tests for neurology.

- In the 1940s, physiologists Hodgkin, Huxley and Eccles demonstrated through intracellular nerve cell recordings the generation of electrical discharges by the sodium/potassium exchange.

- Szent-Gyorgyi, the Nobel laureate who discovered the biologic oxidation mechanism of vitamin C, said "Some basic fact about life is still missing." His concept that solid-state electronic processes were generated by biologic molecules reawakened interest in electrobiology.

- A number of investigators demonstrated major influence of DC current on neuronal behavior and a variety of influences of electricity upon brain function, mood, personality and sleep.

- In 1976, Nias demonstrated in double-blind studies the benefits of electrosleep, which had already been used in the USSR for more than twenty-five years. Electrosleep is one of the great unused electrotherapeutic discoveries of this century.

- Eventually the solid-state electronic activity of the neuron system was proven by Ishiko and Lowenstein's demonstration of potential changes induced by raising temperatures without action potential effects in nerve fibers. These and similar DC changes in the eye cannot be explained on the basis of ion exchanges. And indeed, Libet and Gerard had reported in the 1940s electrical brain current of a non-ionic nature, what today would be called "displacement current." Most brain activity is created by intracellular-to-extracellular (and vice versa) movement of sodium, potassium, calcium, and magnesium ions. Electricity and chemistry are inseparable in living organisms.

- In the 1960s Dr. Robert Becker, an orthopedist, and his coworkers demonstrated that currents of only 30 microamps could induce loss of consciousness and general anesthesia in salamanders. They found that an

electromagnetic field at strengths of 3000 gauss oriented 90 degrees in a fronto-occipital vector produced
similar results. Later experiments demonstrated a magnetic field around the head, with eventual development
of a magnetoencephalogram, the magnetic field of the
brain, as contrasted with the electrical.

Concomitantly, Becker resurrected early 1900 experiments using electrical current to assist in regenerating tissue
regrowth of limbs or tails in salamanders and even of the
forearm. But he was not successful in regenerating the paws
of cats. His work later led to the development of electrical
current that improves healing of fractures of various bones.
Becker believed that intrinsic electromagnetic energy inherent in the nervous system of the body is therefore the factor
that exerts the major controlling influence over growth
processes in general. Indeed, Becker believed electromagnetic
property to be intrinsic in all living tissues.

The Piezoelectronic Connection

Piezoelectric means the ability to convert pressure into electricity. The piezoelectronic property of bone was established
in 1954. The piezoelectric mechanism produces an electrical
stimulus evoked by mechanical stress or pressure. Becker

established the piezoelectrical properties of even collagen, the universal "glue" substance of the body. Dentin, tendon, aorta, trachea, bone, intestines, elastin and nucleic acids are all normal human anatomical transducers of piezoelectro-energy. Thus, we are all living piezoelectric generators!

Carrying this correlation of living tissue to electrical phenomena further, others have demonstrated the electro-magnetic foundation for activity in frog sciatic nerve, growth of bacteria, production of carbon dioxide by yeast, division in sea urchin eggs and in cholates, normal bile salts.

Becker's work with living systems eventually led him to study the association between externally generated electro-magnetic fields and the normal bioelectromagnetics of life itself. Electromagnetic energy activates the piezoelectric property of tissue to emit phonons, sound waves with a wavelength low enough to resonate with cell membranes. Thus, electromagnetism is responsible for the chemical and physical aspects of life itself.

Indeed it is this bioelectromagnetic aspect that is largely responsible for known and unknown biological cycles or clocks, best known as the circadian or diurnal rhythm (variations during night and day or the twenty-four-hour variations).

In 1954, Frank Brown, a scientist at Northwestern

University, demonstrated that oysters that were moved from New Hampshire to Illinois changed the opening and closing of their shells to coincide with the tides at the new location, as if Illinois were a seacoast. Similarly, the night/day timing of many neurochemicals, such as blood levels of cortisol in human beings, change when they are transported great distances longitudinally.

In general, this change is accomplished at a rate of about one hour per day. Thus, a trip from New York to Australia requires at least seven days for a person to accommodate naturally to the new time zone biologically. One of the most critical changes is an individual's production of melatonin, which is essential for good sleep. Jet lag may be the most widely recognized negative effect of electromagnetic distortion in today's fast-paced world. "Artificially" changing one's natural electromagnetic fields by rapidly moving great distances is a twentieth-century development.

During the last thirty years, extensive work has demonstrated that natural electromagnetic phenomena are involved in the migrations of birds, fish and even honeybees. Some bacteria even orient themselves to the earth's magnetic field, apparently because they contain microcrystals of magnetite (the smallest known unit of magnetism). Only recently have similar crystals been found in the human brain. Preliminary research indicates that humans appear to have some electromagnetic tracking sense, which is disrupted when magnets with strengths ranging from 140 to 300 gauss are applied to their heads. Eels tested in the United States are affected by DC electrical fields of 0.67 microvolts/cm and currents of 0.00167 microamps/cm^2, truly subtle influences.[1]

The Influence of Electromagnetic Fields

Central to understanding bioelectromagnetism is the 7 to 10 Hz (cycles per second) frequency that is the dominant rhythm of the earth and a common frequency component of the EEG of all higher animals and humans.

Applied electromagnetic energy can elicit, control or trigger biological changes. Becker emphasized that electromagnetic fields can be stressors. Adrenal production of cortisol, an adrenal hormone essential to life, is significantly altered by pulsed electromagnetic energy. The degree of effect depends on a field's strength and frequency, the duration of exposure (continuous versus intermittent) and even a being's predisposition.

Electromagnetic waves from television, radio, microwaves, radar and satellites bombard us today. These human-made, artificial EMFs overwhelmingly dominate the earth's normal electromagnetic environment, that from the sun! Almost all areas of the world have electric fields of 0.10/m or greater or magnetic ones of 100 microgauss or more. Average exposures may be eight to ten times these fields. In the former Soviet Union, "safe" exposure was felt to be below 1 microwatt/cm^2. We will not know the ultimate epidemiologic health effects of such massive changes in environmental EMFs for many years.

When people are removed from the normal 10 Hz background by placing them in specially shielded rooms, their EEGs, mood and diurnal (day–night) neurochemistry change. The thyroid, pancreas and adrenal glands are all affected by EMFs.

Similarly, cumulative external electromagnetic influences can affect mood, sleep, health and even EEG. We now know that electric blankets are extremely dangerous to the fetus in pregnant women, with marked increases in miscarriage and malformations. In patients who are stressed beyond healthy coping ability and have chronic depression, the EEG shows significant asymmetry, most often including

- Excess activity in the right frontal lobe;
- Inability to follow flickering light frequency;
- Inappropriate EEG, excess speeding up or slowing down with flickering lights;

• Abnormal EEG activity even with an electric clock near the head.

Such individuals sometimes become so sensitive that radio waves may be disturbing to their cognitive congruence.

In Germany, Rutgerin has performed complex experiments on humans in underground, electromagnetically shielded rooms. He has demonstrated that 10 Hz electrical fields assist humans in returning to normal diurnal patterns when they have been destabilized and desynchronized by staying in such shielded rooms.

EEG changes and diurnal rhythms of humans have been induced by a change of magnetism applied for only one to three minutes at 200 to 1,000 gauss as well as EMFs of 3 to 50 Hz. (The magnetic field of the earth is only $1/2$ gauss.) Pulsed EMFs have also been reported to evoke changes in neuronal firing behavior, as well as to effect individual responses to drugs. That is, the threshold for nerve action is lowered and sensitivity to drugs increased. Such effects may occur at levels of EMFs as low as 30 microwatts/cm^2. Remember that an electric light uses 120 volts and consumes 60–150 watts of energy. Even in tissue culture, minute amounts of electromagnetic energy can affect brain tissue production of norepinephrine.

Biological effects can occur at electromagnetic levels well below those of thermal energy. Animals exposed to higher levels of energy, such as 200–300 gauss for seventy hours, show major anatomical damage of brain tissue. Even 60 microwatts/cm^2 of 3 GHz energy applied for up to six weeks causes brain damage.

EMFs can influence the degree of aggression, avoidance patterns and sleep patterns of animals. Pulsed magnetic fields change humans' reaction times. Even 1 gauss of 60 Hz can alter human concentration. Extremely low EMFs of just .00001 volts can alter EEGs.

In nonendocrine tissues, the rhythm of the heart can be easily altered by EMFs. And, at extremely low levels, EMFs of 25 to 50 microwatts/cm^2 can change white blood cells dramatically. Becker concludes, "There is no biological function which can be said to be impervious to non-thermal EMFs—they are a fundamental and pervasive factor in the biology of every living organism."[2]

Meanwhile, beneficial therapeutic effects of applied EMFs are increasing. Perhaps the most pervasive use has been cardiac pacing, where millions of lives have been gratifyingly and effectively prolonged with pacemakers. Pain control, through TENS (transcutaneous electrical nerve stimulator) or electroacupuncture, is also at the forefront of bioelectromagnetic therapy.

THE SECRET OF LIFE

Throughout history, philosophers and mystics have pondered about the energy of life itself. In every culture, except that of modern scientific monotheism, life is considered sacred, the physical manifestation of spiritual energy emanating from a Divine Source. Though the majority of us share common beliefs, science has ignored or suppressed interest in the nature of life itself since the days of René Descartes' infamous statement, "I think; therefore I am."

The concept of *thinking* itself is poorly understood by scientists, religious leaders and laypersons because it defies scientific explanation. The *Random House College Dictionary* defines thinking as 1. rational; reasoning; 2. thoughtful; reflective; studious. In an attempt to make humans the ultimate creation, many scientists have insisted that animals don't think, plan, play or have emotions. This seems hard to believe when you associate with animals and watch their behavior! Ignorance, as Dr. Edward Bach (1886–1936) has defined it, is simply the failure to accept truth. Thinking is one aspect of life but not the basic one—the energy that distinguishes life from inanimate objects.

Energy is the basic framework of the universe, down to individual atoms. Life energy is simply one aspect of consciousness. The effects of consciousness and the *influence* of unseen spiritual energy can be detected electromagnetically.

We can no longer separate relatedness of biochemistry, physical anatomy and electromagnetism. However, the scientific community is slow in altering its perception that physical reality is the only reality.

The medical community is overdue in regarding health as both the well-being and lack of disease in both the human body and its spirit. A model for health should reflect that the human spirit is connected with the body through an electromagnetic field.

The Electromagnetic Framework of Life

Life is considered to include bacteria, fungi and viruses, as well as amoebae, plants, all animals and humans. However, what is the distinction between bacteria and human life? Basically this is *life energy.*

China, the oldest continuous civilization, considers life to be a result of *chi* or *qi.* Chi comes from the universe and flows through the body in channels or acupuncture meridians. A German scientist, Wilhelm Reich (1897–1957), one of the few psychiatrists to consider life energy and study it scientifically, referred to life energy as *orgone.*

A Russian engineer, Georges Lakhovsky (1869–1942), published his book *The Secret of Life* more than seventy years ago in which he emphasized the vibratory frequency of DNA as 50-plus billion cycles per second, or Gigahertz. Modern Ukrainian quantum physicists have taken Lakhovsky's concepts much further and refer to it as the study of Giga-energy. They report that human DNA vibrates at 52 to 78 Gigahertz (billions of cycles per second); animals at 47 Gigahertz; and plants at 42 Gigahertz. They believe that each individual resonates most significantly at a unique, eigen or individual frequency. Thus, there could be 27 billion specific frequencies, from 52 billion cycles per second up to 78.99999 billion cycles per second.

Furthermore, these physicists believe each human organ, because of its anatomic structure, projects its vector, or energy, along a specific pathway for that organ, the acupuncture meridian for that organ. Thus, modern physics is providing a foundation for integrating acupuncture, an ancient wisdom, with quantum theory.

In December 1992, I traveled to the Ukraine to work with these scientists. Those twelve days began my study of Giga-energy. I have been able to confirm many of their findings and believe that this subtle energy, at *one-billionth of a watt per cm²* is the electromagnetic support system for chi.

DHEA Hormone as a Measurement for Healing

I believe we can measure a chemical reflection of chi. Before visiting the Ukraine, I had already been interested in the human hormone DHEA and was intrigued by reports that DHEA declines after age thirty. DHEA manifests from cholesterol, and cholesterol increases in many persons after age thirty. I wondered if a correlation existed between DHEA and cholesterol, perhaps due to an acquired enzyme deficiency.

Since women have virtual total deficiencies of progesterone after menopause, I was curious whether progesterone replacement would enhance DHEA production. Despite lack of scientific evidence that progesterone can convert to DHEA, I proceeded to test my theory on seven men. The results were impressive indeed. In every case, their DHEA significantly increased from 30 percent to 100 percent, with an average increase of 60 percent. I have increasingly been led to believe that DHEA is the chemical battery reflecting one's life energy reservoir.

EMOTIONAL CURES VIA ORGASMIC
BIOELECTRICAL RELEASE

The third most influential psychiatrist in history, Wilhelm Reich, set out to answer whether a sexual orgasm is an essentially mechanical process. Freud considered orgasm to be simply a "mechanical" release. This limited mechanistic view led psychiatrists to conclude it was not natural for women to experience orgasm since they had no mechanical release, or ejaculation!

Reich felt that orgastic potency was the key to understanding emotional life in general and psychic disorders or neuroses in particular. Thus Reich assumed that sexual tension and relaxation require a "bioelectrical discharge" during orgasm.

Reich noted that genital friction led to involuntary genital muscle contracture, greater with gentle, slow friction than vigorous, rapid friction. He believed that strongly muscularly armored (blocked) individuals preferred vigorous movement and were vegetatively inhibited.

Reich claimed that the basic function of all living matter, namely tension and relaxation, charge and discharge, were part of the natural function of orgasm. Thus orgastic bioelectric discharge produced pleasure and relaxation, which when blocked resulted in tension and anxiety and separation from the partner. Thus he considered orgasm "one of the most important modal points of the body–soul problem."[3]

In orgastic function the first requirement is vegetative excitation and increased blood flow to the genitals, a parasympathetic effect, producing increased genital tone. Sympathetic anxious excitation leads to constriction of arteries and decreased blood flow. Thus increased tension during sexual excitation has a direct mechanical basis. But voluntary tensing of the genital muscles impedes gratification.

He noted that the involuntary muscle tension created by genital friction was the same as that created by electrically stimulating muscles. Eventually the friction leads to muscle clonus—involuntary automatic contractions concomitant with orgasm. The mechanical friction and tension builds an electrical charge which must lead to both mechanical and electrical discharge. He insisted that post-orgasmic relaxation was not mechanical but bioelectric.

Thus he considered the normal, natural process of orgasm to be tension → discharge → relaxation, the centerpiece of his concept of expansion/contraction as the governing principle in life itself. Mechanical tension, he determined, led to an electrical discharge, and electrical discharge led to mechanical relaxation. He felt this link between mechanics and electricity was also a distinguishable characteristic of living matter—but of course, piezoelectricity is not necessarily living!

Reich emphasized that the sympathetic system acts like calcium—it produces tension—whereas the parasympathetic system acts like potassium, leading to relaxation. He further believed that cholesterol is like calcium and lecithin like potassium. Alkalines behave like potassium and acids like calcium.

There is an antithesis between sexuality and anxiety—the parasympathetic leads to peripheral excitation and central relaxation of sexual expansion; the sympathetic leads to peripheral relaxation and central excitation or anxiety.

Electrical discharge in muscles leads to mechanical relaxation. As mechanical muscle tension builds, the piezoelectric effect increases the voltage gradient. At some critical gradient electric overload occurs, leading to that electrical discharge.

Sexual arousal is an electrical charging of the erogenous surface (genitals, for example), and orgasm is a discharge of the potential accumulated during stimulation/activation. Thus, Reich concluded that orgasm is a basic manifestation of living substance, and the tension–charge formula cannot be applied to nonliving nature.

Skin response to emotions changes electrical potential and resistance, the electrical function of sexual zones being different from that of the rest of the skin. Sexual skin (genitals, tongue, lips, nipples, ears) have other much higher or lower potential than nonsexual skin. "Muscular motor activity in general and rhythmic friction, the rubbing together of pleasurably excitable body surfaces, are the fundamental biological phenomena of sexuality."[4] Friction without plea-sure does not increase potential. Friction with pleasure does. In anxiety or annoyance, surface potential decreases.

Reich believed that the vegetative muscle system is the generator of bioelectrical energy in the human body. Since sexually responsive skin is the only skin that responds with marked increase in potential, he concluded that sexual activity is the bioenergetic productive process itself.

Obviously, all muscle tension is part of the total bioelec-trical energy system. Is it possible that electromagnetic therapy and sacred healing affect the same pathways? Because electromagnetism is such an important part of life, I wish to discuss a few electromagnetic therapies. The devices mentioned here are all safe and well within U.S. government safety guidelines. Their potential benefits seem so great, in many instances, that it appears wise to consider using them. First, it's important to know about early-twenty-first-cen-tury concepts about electromagnetic therapy.

ACUPUNCTURE:
AN ANCIENT EMT TECHNIQUE

Acupuncture is the oldest known form of energetic medicine. Amazingly, there is more valid scientific proof of its effectiveness than any other nonconventional therapy. Acupuncture may be considered the foundation for an understanding of electromagnetic principles in healing.

Although acupuncture has flourished in China for 4,000 years, modern Western medicine rejected it until recently. Interestingly, Sir William Osler considered acupuncture the "treatment of preference" in lumbago (low back pain) as late as 1912. Personally I have used it for more than thirty years to treat pain and many other symptoms.

Dr. Robert Becker, exploring the body's semiconductive capabilities, demonstrated that the tissues around nerves were such semiconductors. He postulated that acupuncture points were areas of amplifier boosters built along transmission cables to propagate electrical signals. Many other investigators have shown that acupuncture points have lower electric resistance than nonacupuncture points. Pomeranz showed that acupunctured points had injury current as high as 10 microamps and this current's injury lasts several days. Dr. William Tiller, Stanford University professor of materials science, postulates there is a magnetic field above acupuncture channels that creates a battery-like effect at acupuncture points with increased electrical conductivity. This battery would then represent part of a complex electrical system emanating from individual organs. Ukrainian nuclear physicists postulate such a vector system. For instance, heart DNA cells resonate at 52 to 78 billion cycles per second and radiate a vector along specific pathways (meridians) to the tips of the fingers or toes, with a resonating circuit back to the organ. Dr. Hans Popp, a German scientist, believes there are many charged oscillators in the body that send out a variety of electromagnetic waves, some of which are emitted from the body. Dr. Nordstrom, a Swedish physician, postulates that living electrical circuits travel in the fascial tissue around blood vessels, as well as interconnecting with the electrical circuits of nerves.

Acupuncture Principles

Acupuncture meridians are located near the surface of the body between muscle groups. Acupuncture points lie in the depressions between muscle groups. The points coexist with deeper muscle–nerve points (the actual nerve interface with the muscle) 75 percent of the time.

Acupuncture needles are stainless steel with a contrasting metal handle. This bimetallic effect is one of three mechanisms that make acupuncture an inherent electrical treatment. When two different metals are placed in a salt solution, a current flow is created by the different electrical conductivity of the two metals. Secondly, the tip of the needle in the body is warmer than the handle (perhaps 25°F or greater), creating an electrical gradient. The spiral handle is a radiator, proving a larger surface area than the tip. Electrons transfer from one metal to the next as needle temperature varies and the handle oxidizes.

The tip of the needle becomes positive relative to the handle. If the handle is heated or manually twirled, the tip becomes negative, providing additional electrical flow. It takes sixty to ninety minutes for such flow to reach equilibrium. Two needles physically separated in the body on two different acupuncture points thus electrically connect by an electron wave from the twirling, heated or electrically stimulated needle to a stable needle not manipulated.

Ancient Chinese did not understand or describe electrical circuits. They talked about a life force circulating in the body's meridians to protect, nourish and animate all life, generating warmth and stimulating all bodily functions and organs. Such a concept is universal. Ancient Greeks called it "pneuma"; eastern Indians "prana"; Paracelsus called it "quintessence"; Galvani labeled it "animal electricity"; Hahnemann, father of homeopathy, referred to it as the "vital force"; and Mesmer "magnetism." Modern medicine uses only "vitality" but has no concept of a circuit for this vitality.

Modern studies of acupuncture's benefits include the following:

- Improvement in PMS (premenstrual syndrome) with treatment of the sexual circuit (Tchong Mo).
- Restoration of fertility in two-thirds of infertile men through treatment of the Tchong Mo circuit. One man increased his sperm count from 9 to 54 million (a 600 percent increase), which had not been accomplished with any modern medical approach.[5]
- Control of migraine in approximately three-quarters of patients.
- Restoration of DHEA (dehydroepiandrosterone) in two-thirds of individuals.

Chinese divide qi or chi into Wei Qi, Rong Qi, and Yuan Qi. Wei Qi is produced by digestion and internal organ metabolism. It is said to surround the body like a shield, preventing environmental forces from affecting the inner channels. Wei Qi controls sweating, warmth and integrity of the skin and superficial fascia.

Rong Qi is the end product of the total vitality received from food and drink, mixed with inhaled air. Rong Qi circulates with blood inside the body as well as in the energy channels that link organs with the surface of the body. Rong Qi is both the result of and essential to balanced functioning of the internal organs.

Original energy, Yuan Qi, is the genetic, inherited, constitutional energetic component. It is the precursor of all other qi, is *not* reversible and is responsible for growth, development, reproduction, transformation and aging. It resides in the kidney and circulates through extra channels that regulate or balance all energy in the body. Since it cannot be replaced, Yuan Qi is greatly respected, as it can be depleted by physical, mental, emotional or sexual exhaustion or unwise diet.

The twelve meridians are the principal circuits for energy circulation. They allow qi, or vital energy, to move constantly. Acupuncture needles are used to activate the circuits, adding or subtracting energy to balance deficient or excess energy in any organ.

In one sense, the Chinese expressed the essence of electrical "charge" with their concept of yin and yang, negative and positive. Chinese cosmology also includes descriptions of elements. These are wood (flexibility, relatively yang), fire (brilliance, passion, yang), earth (solidity, balanced yin/yang), metal (structural integrity, relatively yin) and water (fluidity, yin).

According to acupuncture's principles

- Kidney, a yang organ, manages water, osmotic regulation and fluid excretion (totally compatible with modern medicine). It also is associated with adrenal and sexual function.
- Heart, a yin organ, not only pumps blood but energetically expresses spirit and creativity, a widespread metaphysical concept.
- Small intestine is responsible for digestion and absorption of food and liquid (same for modern medicine).
- Bladder regulates the elimination of fluid (as in modern medicine) and partially controls the central nervous system, along with the kidney. (The latter is an interesting analogy, since brain function is so remarkably related to cerebrospinal fluid production, absorption and circulation.)
- Liver and gallbladder are "wood" organs. Certainly the liver is the most flexible of all organs.
- Master of the Heart (sympathetic system) and Triple Master are "fire organs," and nothing is more synchronous with the fire of the body than the autonomic nervous system, which includes adrenalin, the "fire" chemical for reaction to stress.

- Stomach (earth) and large intestine (metal) involve all aspects of digestion, just as in modern medicine.
- Spleen (earth) is concerned with blood (as in modern medicine) and includes pancreatic function in Chinese energetics.
- Lung (metal) includes respiration.
- Skin is considered an organ of respiration, which, when we consider sweating, is not too far-fetched in modern Western terms.

In summary, acupuncture is an ancient technique for activation of the electromagnetic system. Insertion of a metal needle into a chemical reservoir, the body, generates a flow of electricity. This fact can be proven. Beyond that, the effects of acupuncture may be a subtle form of sacred healing.

ELECTROMAGNETIC DYSTHYMIA: A UNIVERSAL ILLNESS IN NEED OF HEALING

A dazzling array of symptoms of illnesses may collectively be referred to as Electromagnetic Dysthymia (EMD). To some extent I consider EMD to be a spiritual or existential illness. Perhaps EMD represents the most common illness affecting humanity. It has been totally mystifying to the medical community.

Every illness will eventually overload and weaken the adrenal glands, which ordinarily balance the body's stress level. Thus, adrenal burnout, a prominent cause of EMD, is also involved in every major disease. As long as the body can restore homeostasis or natural balance, major disease does not occur and DHEA levels remain reasonably adequate. As adrenal capability fails, DHEA progressively declines, weakening the immune system and reducing one's total life energy.

How does EMD relate to the great diseases of modern society, heart disease, cancer, stroke, diabetes and others? Stress is the cumulative pressure that we encounter in going about our daily lives:

- Physical—fractures, cuts, excess cold or hot
- Chemical—alcohol, nicotine, caffeine, food additives
- Electromagnetic—radio, TV, computers, enzymes
- Mental—worry, frustration
- Emotional—fear, guilt, anger, anxiety, depression
- Spiritual—moral issues, existential questions

Illness is the body's reaction to total life stress. If EMD manifests burnout or overload of the body's electromagnetic framework, the primary factor being stress, then other illnesses represent overload in the organ system(s) most involved. In EMD, the crisis is a spiritual or existential one.

For instance, in the case of coronary artery disease, the dominant influencing factor is unresolved anger that blocks forgiveness, compassion, love and ultimately the very life force (in this case blood) to the heart itself. A stroke is the failure to use reason and/or wisdom. In diabetes, the body's conflict is related to resentment over having too much or too little. Cancer is virtually always the end result of intense depression, secondarily focused on the organ or body part involved. For instance, breast cancer represents depression over a perception of inadequate nurturing. Prostate or uterine cancer involves problems of security and/or sexuality.

And so it goes. Fear, anxiety, resentment, anger, guilt and depression block life energy. The electromagnetic deprivation of energy impacts the organ or body region with the greatest unresolved emotional distress.

Diagnosing EMD

The Cornell Medical Index (CMI) was touted a generation ago as adequate for making a clinical diagnosis with 80 percent accuracy, without any need for a person to undergo physical examination or lab tests. The CMI includes family history and past history.

The manifestation of thirty or more symptoms in one person in one year indicates the beginning of the body's failure to cope adequately with stress. Of course, thirty-plus symptoms might be present in a serious illness such as cancer or psychosis, so careful diagnostic testing is required to rule out other treatable illnesses.

The list of EMD symptoms overall describes adrenal exhaustion and liver and heart muscle dysfunction according to the Grand Master Healer Ostad Hadi Parvarandeh. EMD symptoms include the following:

- Chronic fatigue
- Immune system problems
- Depression
- Lowered DHEA
- Intracellular magnesium deficiency
- Deficiency of one or more essential amino acids
- EEG brain map abnormalities

These are symptoms of many chronic illnesses. Ultimately EMD is diagnosed when every usual physical illness is ruled out.

Chronic Fatigue Syndrome

Chronic Fatigue Syndrome is simply one extreme of EMD. The illness typifies EMD, as it relates to stress overload of the adrenal glands. One of the more controversial illnesses of the last decade, the syndrome appears to have existed in the 1800s and was referred to as "neurasthenia." Florence Nightingale probably suffered from it. Other diagnoses have also been used to describe this confusing array of symptoms, including Wilson's disease, chronic Epstein-Barr, candidiasis, environmental sensitivity and myeloencephalopathy.

The prominent symptoms of Chronic Fatigue Syndrome are lack of energy, poor quality sleep, a need for more sleep or rest than normal, anxiety, irritability and weakness. No specific diagnostic test exists for these symptoms. Many treatments produce only transient improvement, if any.

Most of these individuals have probably experienced a major life crisis, such as divorce, that initiated a progressive dis-ease and perhaps a situational depressive reaction. However, some individuals with this condition have never felt happy. Thus, it seems Chronic Fatigue Syndrome may be a disease of the spirit.

The Link Between Hormonal and
Nutritional Deficiencies and EMD

Although much of the medical literature states true dehydroepiandrosterone (DHEA) deficiency is a diagnosis for men with less than 180 mg/dL and for women with less than 130 mg/dL, DHEA levels below each gender's mean (715 in men and 510 in women) imply progressively diminished adrenal reserve. Most patients with EMD have levels less than 50 percent of the mean, and none have levels at the mean or above. Therefore, DHEA deficiency is common and present in virtually every major illness, as well as in EMD, suggesting relative adrenal exhaustion or adrenal maladaptation.

Magnesium regulates membrane potential, the resting electrical charge on cells. A deficiency of magnesium contributes considerably to the increased sensitivity of patients with EMD. Eighty percent of women and 70 percent of men do not consume the recommended daily intake of magnesium, which is usually obtained from eating appropriate amounts of fruits and veggies. Rampant magnesium deficiency is associated with most chronic illnesses. Though low intracellular magnesium is not diagnostic of any disease, EMD is inevitably associated with such deficiency.

Malnutrition is also common in many chronic illnesses,

particularly in chronically depressed patients. The body's essential amino acids produce most of our neurochemicals. Thus, norepinephrine, serotonin, melatonin and beta-endorphin—all crucial neurochemicals essential for feeling energetic—cannot be properly balanced when there is a deficiency in the amino acid building blocks.

Taurine is now considered an essential amino acid by many scientists. It is deficient in 86 percent of patients with depression. The deficiency of both magnesium and taurine evokes hypersensitivity in patients with EMD. Thus, they have a lower tolerance for many stressors.

THE BEGINNING OF A CURE

The EMD malady is much more common than any other disease and indeed is concomitant in many diseases. In its simplest form, EMD results in significant depression. As an individual's ability to cope with increasing stress—including noise, poor nutrition, psychosocial pressures and pollution—is lost, homeostasis becomes erratic and DHEA begins to decrease.

I spoke earlier about how electromagnetic pollution increasingly contributes to stress. Fluorescent lights, electrical appliances and devices, automobiles, airplanes, radio and

TV waves and radar all bombard the human energy system daily. This may provide major electromagnetic stress, which appears to lead to an ever-increasing incidence of depression and EMD.

Sir William Osler's belief that there is one common cause of illness may be correct. We should accept that depression and various stress illnesses indicate an electromagnetic (psychoneuroimmunologic) overload. There is evidence to prove EMD results from chemical, physical, emotional and electromagnetic stress on the body, which affects the limbic system and hypothalamus, leading to a loss of electrical homeostasis of the brain/mind. EMD illness manifests as depression, with or without a multiple system disease.

The major stress-reduction techniques listed below provide the foundation for therapy. Eighty-five percent of patients respond initially to two weeks of intensive multimodal treatment, and 70 percent improve long-term.

- Photostimulation
- Education
- Music
- Biofeedback
- Guided imagery
- Autogenic training

Recovery may be assisted by magnesium replacement and amino acid supplementation, DHEA restoration and use of the Liss TENS devices transcranially.

A number of letters from patients with chronic fatigue or depression attest that they consider themselves healed after being treated by sacred healers. Because EMD is a disease primarily of low vital energy, I have to consider it the prime example of a spiritual dis-ease and thereby one that might benefit from sacred healing practices.

10

Holy Water— Sacred Water

I have referred briefly to ancient healing springs and holy water, as well as water in which the hydrogen bonding has been changed by healers such as Olga Worrall. As this book is going to press, I am tremendously impressed and enthusiastic about a unique liquid that has been discovered by a fellow Sagittarian, Jim Carter, whom I consider a wizard.

We all know that after air, water is the most essential element for life. All food and the vast majority of the human body is made of water. Suppose there is another liquid so similar to common water or mixed with common water that it cannot be easily distinguished.

The book of Genesis implies that the world was created from the void and that water was the "mother liquor." To this water was added the Logos, or the "Word of God," producing many substances or many waters. The importance of water for both cleansing the physical body and for spiritual cleansing was established, with the baptism of Christ; this act of healing or "washing away sins" is the foundation for Christianity.

In the late 1800s and at least up until the 1940s, healing springs all over the world were extremely popular. In 1870 Doug Tyrell, a world-renowned physician, wrote a book entitled *The Royal Road to Health*. One chapter was "The Cure for all Disease," and the remedy he wrote of was water. The glacial waters the Hunzas drink are said to be the secret of their longevity.

The search for Magic Water or the Fountain of Youth is one of humanity's oldest quests. When I first encountered this unusual material that in some cases looks and acts like oil and in others looks like and mixes with water, I was extremely impressed. I spent an afternoon talking with the discoverer of this unique product, rubbing the material on my hands and face and feeling increasingly energized. Afterwards, my appetite was pleasantly diminished and during the next couple of days I ate less than half my usual intake of food. I took a bath in a large tub of warm water with only two ounces of this unusual oil/water material. It was extremely energizing. I slept on a bed of crystal resembling sand with lots of mica in it, which is one of the sources of this material. When I awoke the following morning, my tinnitus of eight years' duration was gone.

Since that time, I have continued to use this water/oil, which I will call Sacred Water, rubbing about one ounce per day on my body or putting two ounces per day in a hot tub of water for a soak. This eliminates my tinnitus at least 50 percent of the time. When I also sleep on a pillow of the mica-crystal, my tinnitus is virtually nonexistant throughout the day.

A number of people also report tremendous anecdotal benefits from this Sacred Water. A man, after six weeks of using it, was able to stop taking anti-hypertensive medication and has remained off medication for the next several months. A woman lost sixty-five pounds in eight months without dieting and markedly improved her energy and her mood. Her hair turned from gray to mostly red with only a few streaks of gray. She now looks twenty years younger than she did eight months ago. There is no sagging of skin from her rapid weight loss.

I was so impressed with this Sacred Water that I tested it on fifty of my students who had had their DHEA electively measured earlier. We gave them enough Sacred Water to use two ounces per day in a tub in which thay were to soak for twenty minutes. At the end of eight days, their DHEA was redrawn. In all but two of the students, the DHEA went down 40 to 60 percent!

I have only previously heard of such an unusual drop in DHEA one other time: When Ostad did his initial healing. Despite the lowering of DHEA, many people reported increased energy, elimination of allergy and weight loss of as much as seven pounds in eight days.

I have discussed this material with the three most outstanding intuitives I know. Independently, each of them agrees this material that looks like oil and acts like water is unique and has the power to significantly reverse the aging process, restore function to many parts of the body and reduce arthritic pain. This Sacred Water acts like a lubricant. It seems to detoxify the body. Perhaps it works by transferring the subtle etheric energy body directly into the physical body, acting as a major catalyst, and it may be using DHEA in its process of detoxifying and rejuvenating the body. Studies are under way to test whether over a three- to six-month period the DHEA in my test subjects will not only return to its initial value but keep increasing as these people continue to improve symptomatically.

Super Water, Holy Water, Sacred Water. We may well be on the verge of discovering the Fountain of Youth.

11

Electrotherapy
for Healing

I believe sacred healers tap into cosmic energy, or chi. I also believe we can to some extent activate the body's chi with electrotherapy.

Electrotherapy has intrigued naturalist physicians for almost 2,000 years. In 46 A.D., Scribonius Largus described how an electric ray was used to treat both headaches and painful gout. In the late nineteenth and early twentieth centuries, electrotherapy peaked in popularity. It was claimed to cure virtually every conceivable symptom or illness. The Bakken Library in Minneapolis has a magnificent collection of devices, some as large as a room, all claiming in their day to cure virtually everything.

ELECTROTHERAPY DEVICES

The Electreat

Ultimately, only one of the popular devices survived the witch hunt of the Flexner Report: the Electreat, patented in 1919 by C. W. Kent, a naturopath from Peoria, Illinois. The device remained on the market in the 1940s, despite intense attack by the FDA and rejection by the medical profession.

In 1951, my father suffered painful facial paralysis, Bell's palsy. Unsuccessfully treated by several physicians, he consulted a chiropractor who prescribed an Electreat, which provided relief from pain and full recovery. In 1960, when I had neck and arm pain from a ruptured cervical disc, my father gave me his Electreat. Because of its somewhat clumsy design and my lack of insight into its potential, unfortunately, I barely used it. However, I was impressed by the many claims of its curative power and the machine's peculiar ability to pass an electrical current from one person to another.

Then, a seemingly inconsequential event occurred in 1963. Dr. William Collins, a neurosurgeon, left Western Reserve where both of us were on faculty and moved to Virginia. He had begun studying pain physiology before I arrived at the university. As a joke, I presented him with the

Electreat at his going-away party. We laughed at the internal electrode and the electric comb as superstition or snake oil.

In 1965, when Pat Wall introduced his concept of the spinal gate as the physiological mechanism for pain, I remembered the Electreat. (Basically Drs. Wall and Melzack at MIT demonstrated that the smallest "C" nerve fibers enter the spinal cord with pain information and may there be blocked by input over the largest Beta fibers, which modulate or regulate pain input. This "gate" also can be closed by descending fibers from the brain.) By that time, Bill Collins had discarded my gift. Fortunately, the company was still producing the Electreat in Peoria, and I was able to acquire one.

The Dorsal Column Stimulator

In 1965, I introduced my concept of dorsal column stimulation, proving the value of electrical stimulation of the spinal cord's dorsal columns to suppress pain. In April 1967, modern electrotherapy became a reality. I surgically implanted a battery-powered Dorsal Column Stimulator (DCS) into a man who was terminally ill with widespread cancer; his pain was totally controlled.

Dorsal column stimulation worked well over the next eight years in 75 percent of my patients with chronic pain.

Alas, there are risks involved, and the long-term benefits are not significant enough for me to recommend it to most patients with noncancer pain.

Meanwhile, however, nonsurgical tools have been developed that are equally effective in masking chronic pain in at least 85 percent of patients.

The First Modern TENS

I continued to use the Electreat in my practice. At first, I used it to demonstrate the feeling of electrical stimulation to patients who were to receive a DCS. Later, it was used in treatment. From the outset of my electrotherapy study, I was convinced that external surface or skin stimulation would be applicable at least 1,000 times as often as dorsal column stimulation.

As early as 1967, I had encouraged Medtronic design engineers, who had manufactured my Dorsal Column Stimulator, to produce a modern solid-state Electreat. Medtronic refused because they focused on implantation (they were the originators of cardiac pacemakers).

In the early 1970s, Norman Hagfors, a Medtronic design engineer who had worked on my invention, left Medtronic to establish a new company, Stim-Tech, Inc. Before long, he purchased the Electreat Company and moved it to

Minnesota. The Electreat continued to be manufactured until 1993. Stim-Tech introduced the first solid-state modern skin stimulator, Stim-Tech. The initial, rather large box (approximately a foot square and four inches thick) emitted a pulsed, square wave. I felt this could not be as effective as the spike-type pulsed waves of the Electreat, and with my urging, Medtronic produced a much smaller device with a spiked wave.

In the two decades since the introduction of this early device, a plethora of TENS (Transcutaneous Electrical Nerve Stimulator) devices flooded the market. However, they never penetrated mass-market consciousness or received a single marketing "push" from a pharmaceutical company. Today, Empi is the major producer of TENS.

This year, an estimated 100,000 TENS units will be sold at a projected annual revenue of $100 million. TENS devices relieve approximately 50 percent of chronic pain adequately. Of the 50 million sufferers in this country, probably only 2 percent have chosen this treatment—the safest pain reliever ever introduced.

I had always insisted that modern TENS machines could not measure up to the effectiveness of an Electreat. Though their pulsations were often somewhat more pleasant, the waves neither penetrated nor traveled nearly as extensively through the body. The whole picture became apparent only in 1994, after I discovered GigaTENS. Now more than thirty years after my initial request, I have been able to redesign a device that puts out the frequencies of the old Electreat but in a modern package with modern electrodes and controls. The Shealy TENS is the first device I've allowed to use my name. In one sense I believe the energy of the Shealy TENS comes as close as we can to tapping universal cosmic energy for human use.

Cranial Electrical Stimulation

In 1975, before the FDA placed restrictions on medical devices, Dr. Saul Liss, a medical engineer, introduced his TENS device. Initially called the Pain Suppressor, it was later redesigned and renamed the Liss Body Stimulator. The machine did not impress me on first try because it emitted only 4 milliamps of current, which generally is lower than sensory perception. When Saul made me a 10 milliamp unit, though, I had to admit it was too strong.

By chance, I touched one of the electrodes to my forehead about 10:30 one night. For the next hour, I experimented with the sensation of flickering lights it had evoked. No matter where on the cranial vault one or both of the electrodes were placed, I saw a visual flicker. The flicker was there even with one electrode on top of my head and the other on my foot.

I went to bed about 11:30 P.M. and awoke at 2:30 A.M., unable to sleep any longer because of marked increased energy and alertness. A few months later my associate, Dr. James Kwako, and I both applied this device transcranially at 8:00 A.M. for forty-five minutes. Four hours later my blood serotonin level had increased to five times the upper limit of normal, and Jim's had doubled.

Jim and I decided to try Saul's device on patients with depression. The first patient had been depressed for sixteen years. Remarkably, an hour of transcranial stimulation completely relieved his depression in just one day. Unfortunately, he insisted on returning home to Florida with no more treatments; within one week, his depression returned.

Two findings—serotonin elevation and relief of depression—motivated me to study further. (Serotonin is one of the body's most important neurochemicals, involved in mood regulation, sleep and pain. Serotonin-modulating drugs have been extensively studied for treatment of depression, as well as for migraine headaches.) In seventy-five patients with chronic pain who were given a CES treatment, serotonin output was normalized in 80 percent of them. Of these patients, 40 percent previously had deficient serotonin, and

40 percent had excessive serotonin. One hour of CES treatment daily for two weeks improved their moods and stabilized their serotonin levels.

I had determined that when the Liss unit was used transcranially, it relieved depression in 50 percent of chronically depressed patients who had failed to respond earlier to one or more antidepressant drugs. More recently, we have found that photostimulation, education and vibratory music also relieve depression in 58 percent of chronically depressed patients. But when we combine the two approaches, using CES along with photostimulation, education and vibratory music, a striking 85 percent of patients come out of depression. With no further therapy, 70 percent remain free of depression three to six months later. At this point, we recommend continued use of the CES once or twice a week after the initial daily treatment program.

The Liss device used transcranially is also remarkably helpful in treating insomnia and in overcoming jet lag. It has enhancing effects on beta endorphin, the natural "feel good" narcotic, as well as upon serotonin. There may be a variety of other uses as well. We will talk later about enhancement of DHEA, dehydroepiandrosterone, when the Liss is applied to a specific pattern of acupuncture points.

Ultrasafe, I believe every household should have a TENS

device. Unfortunately, purchase of a TENS requires a pre-scription. Most physicians know virtually nothing about the benefits this device can provide. Because no pharmaceutical company sponsors the TENS, it is likely to continue to be underused unless patients insist that their physicians prescribe it.

GigaTENS

In December 1992, Saul Liss and I were invited to visit Kiev, in the Ukraine, to study a device called the MRT (Microwave Resonance Therapy). According to the hosting quantum physicists, they had discovered this approach twelve years earlier. They said they had learned

- Human DNA resonates at 52 to 78 billion cycles-per-second (gigahertz);
- Animal DNA resonates at 47 gigahertz;
- Plant DNA resonates at 42 gigahertz.

Furthermore, they reported curing 50 percent of narcotic addicts, 92 percent of alcoholics, and more than 80 percent of patients with rheumatoid arthritis when applying 52 to 78 gigahertz at one-billionth of a watt to selected acupuncture points. More than 200,000 patients had been treated with the MRT. Therapy usually lasted a total of thirty minutes per day, five days per week, for two weeks, with remission or a cure occurring for up to two years.

The physicians were treating virtually every illness with MRT, from angina pectoris to diabetes to osteomyelitis (chronic infections of bone). No complications from this therapy were reported.

Liss and I, working with two Ukrainian physicists, redesigned the device to use in several clinical situations. We call the device the GigaTENS and have verified this technology's benefits. Striking pain relief is realized in 70 percent of patients with rheumatoid arthritis for whom conventional drug therapy fails. Pain relief and some neurological improvement are seen in 80 percent of patients with diabetic neuropathy. GigaTENS improves 50 percent of patients with chronic back pain or depression. GigaTENS therapy appears to be the most versatile, safe and effective therapy known to date.

Now that equipment to test giga-frequencies was available, in the summer of 1994, I tested my old favorite, the Electreat. It became clear why I have always preferred the Electreat—it puts out giga-frequency. Amazingly, C. W. Kent had marketed a prototype of GigaTENS in 1919. Considering the experience of the Ukrainian physicians, perhaps

Dr. Kent was right in some of his elaborate claims—it may be the closest thing to a panacea yet.

Dr. William Tiller, a Stanford University materials scientist, and I have now created a smaller, much more user-friendly device, the Shealy TENS, which has all the advantages of TENS plus the superior benefits of giga-frequency. At this point, the Shealy TENS is the safest, most effective stimulator available, the best remedy we know for treatment of pain, depression, insomnia, jet lag, migraine, rheumatoid arthritis and diabetic neuropathy. For pain alone, this device is invaluable. Totally safe, it can be used by virtually everyone except perhaps patients with cardiac pacemakers as the device might interfere with the function of the pacemaker.

Much progress is yet to be made as new types of electromagnetic stimulators and possibly new applications for this type of device evolve. The Electreat was here at the start of the twentieth century. After more than eighty years, it still is more useful than some other modern TENS devices. The Shealy TENS and Liss device are the first known electrotherapy devices that strikingly alter human neurochemistry. These two devices are the foundation for twenty-first-century energy medicine.

Electroacupuncture

When I began dorsal column stimulation in 1967, I inserted needles into the painful areas on patients' bodies and attached electrical stimulators to them. The importance of inserting the needle into the center of pain soon became apparent. This is a rule in classic acupuncture. By the late 1960s, I was calling my technique PENS (Percutaneous Electrical Nerve Stimulation).

Other than having read a bit of literature about it, I had no formal training in acupuncture. In 1973, I went to England to study with Dr. Felix Mann, a British physician who had trained in France and China and translated several ancient acupuncture texts into English. (Mann ordinarily did not use electrical stimulation of acupuncture needles.)

The Chinese knew about my clinic and my work with electrical stimulation, and the first Chinese medical delegation to come to the U.S. after relations with China opened requested to visit me in late 1973. I learned during that visit that the Chinese had begun applying electrical stimulation to acupuncture needles in 1967—the same year I did.

Most Western practitioners now use electrical stimulation for many acupuncture treatments. It has been shown that stimuli at 1 Hz, 1 cycle per second, raises beta endorphin. Higher frequencies, although they may effectively relieve pain, do not raise beta endorphin. Acupuncture, with or without electrical stimulation, does affect cortisol and ACTH (adrenocorticotrophic hormone). Acupuncture also restores fertility in two out of three infertile males, something no known conventional medical treatment can accomplish.

A number of electrical innovations today attempt to capitalize on electroacupuncture. Many do not use needles but just apply focal shocks to acupuncture points. Little scientific study has been done of these techniques or of lasers applied to acupuncture points.

ELECTROMAGNETIC CHARACTERISTICS OF HEALING

Ostad and I used the EEG and EKG during our evaluations because the brain has the software program for the body. Ostad believes it controls every bodily function. The fact that this master healer is able to affect a patient's EEG in a room one hundred feet or more away indicates his energy can access a person's energetic software. He can do the same with EKG and cardiac output. One of Ostad's reports attests that he sent healing energy to a patient in a deep coma at a great distance, and simultaneously the patient's EEG showed activity associated with the healing process.

We decided that it would be appropriate to see what effect Ostad's healing could have on EEG results. A regular EEG is not nearly as easy to read as we in this field have been led to believe. In the waking state, with eyes open, the brain's dominant wave activity is believed to be in the frequency called beta, or 13 to 26 cycles per second. When the eyes are closed, there is an increase in most people's wave cycles of alpha frequency (8 to 12 cycles per second). During daydreaming or creative imagery or visualization, the rhythm of the brain has a modest to sometimes marked increase in theta frequency (4 to 7 cycles per second). Generally, delta frequency (1 to 3 cycles per second) is thought to be present only briefly when individuals are falling asleep. It may also be present locally in damaged areas of the brain. Examples in this book of testing Ostad's sacred healing show the standard EEG recording of an individual who has been resting with eyes closed for several minutes.

A second standard EEG is taken at the exact instant when an individual has had distant healing by Ostad.

A third EEG shows the natural brain wave when Ostad's intent has been to alter the occipital area of the brain.

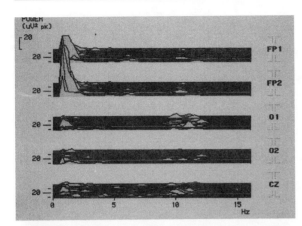

*Baseline
pre-healing.*

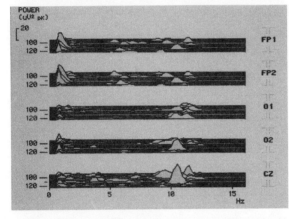

*Note
increased 6
to 12 cycle
frontal activi-
ty in addition
to 10 to 12
cycle central
and occipital
activity.*

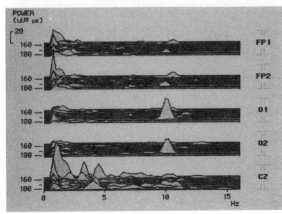

*Note marked
increase in 1
to 15 cycle
centrally and
10 to 11 cycle
occipital
activity.*

FP1 = left front parietal
FP2 = right front parietal
CZ = central
O1 = left occipital
O2 = right occipital

A computerized analysis of the basic brain wave patterns reveals both in the absolute power and the relative power of the basic frequencies.

Another computerized analysis demonstrates both the magnitude in a line graph as well as the magnitude in microvolts as a percentage of power present in the frontal, occipital or central areas of the brain in relation to the same basic patterns.

When you look at this as the cycles per second, it is obvious that in most individuals the strongest activity is actually in the delta range, and the next strongest in usually the low theta range. The computer picks out activity that is not generally noticed by the average visual reading of standard EEG.

In our testing of the first thirty individuals, we asked Ostad, who was sitting in a separate room approximately forty feet away from the patient, to apply his intent to heal only to the front or the back of the patient, without specifying what frequency might be used. Ostad had a full-length polaroid photograph of the individual he was working on, taken both from the front and the rear. We synchronized timing so that the EEG technician could mark the record appropriately at exactly the moment when healing was to occur. The patient had no knowledge whatsoever of when healing would be applied or for how long. Generally the healing was applied for a maximum of two minutes. In those first thirty patients it was two minutes to the frontal area and two minutes to the occipital area, although we alternated whether Ostad applied the energy first occipitally or first frontally.

In tests with another thirty-two patients, we asked Ostad specifically to increase the 10-cycle-per-second, or mid-alpha range frequencies, in either the frontal or occipital part of the brain. The patients were well over one hundred feet away in a totally different building, and the timing was done by synchronized stopwatches.

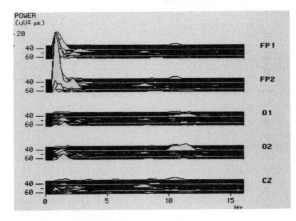

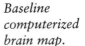

Baseline computerized brain map.

FPI = left front parietal
FP2 = right front parietal
CZ = central
OI = left occipital
O2 = right occipital

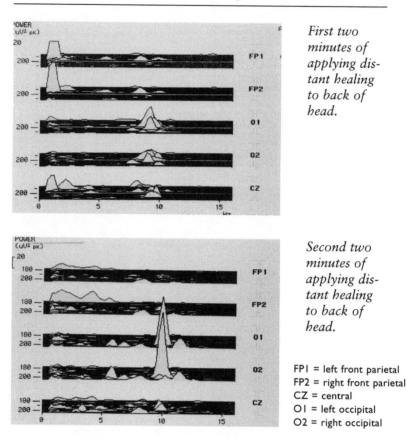

First two minutes of applying distant healing to back of head.

Second two minutes of applying distant healing to back of head.

FPI = left front parietal
FP2 = right front parietal
CZ = central
OI = left occipital
O2 = right occipital

The results are quite striking. When we look at the broad band of alpha, we see almost invariably a decrease in the total power in the alpha range in 88 percent of the patients when Ostad applied healing to the frontal areas and in 80 percent when he applied it to the occipital area. Interestingly, when we look at the power collage, we see that in half of the patients there was no major activity at 10 cycles per second, either before or during healing. But in half of the patients, even though the broad band of the alpha wave had diminished—sometimes quite significantly—in more than 75 percent, there was a marked increase specifically at 10 cycles per second. Interestingly, there was often a much greater change in the center of the brain than in either the occipital or the frontal areas.

Because we did many long periods of control with these EEGs and because these changes took place specifically while Ostad was "sending healing," there is no scientific doubt that somehow he energetically affected the EEG of these individuals. Even in those individuals where there was no measurable change in the 10-cycle activity, it would appear that he still had some overall effect because the total power in the alpha range went down in those individuals. It's as if the 10-cycle borrowed from the rest of the alpha range in order to have that increase occur.

There are two other experiments of energetic effects, one involving the heart. We have equipment that noninvasively measures stroke volume and cardiac output, a very elegant EKG and related computerized equipment developed by Dr. Robert Eliot, a well-known cardiologist who also created the concept of the "hot reactor." In a test of five individuals, again with Ostad positioned more than a hundred feet away in a different room, he was asked to increase cardiac output and stroke volume. There was indeed a marked change in this particular physiological measurement. In the case of the EEG and of the cardiac output, Ostad did not physically touch the patients during the application of healing energy. In the test of the DHEA, he applied his healing hands to patients in sessions that lasted fifteen to twenty minutes per patient.

In a totally nonphysiological testing of his effect on the molecular structure of water, Ostad applied his hands to fifteen sealed plastic bottles of spring water purchased at a regular department store. Fifteen control bottles were sent away for testing to three different sites for infrared absorption and ultraviolet absorption measures before he applied his healing touch to the next fifteen bottles of water. One week later the "treated" water was sent for infrared absorption measurements, five bottles each to three separate sites. Here we have to rely on the interpretation of physicists, but basically it appears that Ostad's healing energy significantly affected the molecular structure of water, because infrared absorption has to do exactly with the hydrogen bonding in water.

Thus, we have four scientific measurements that show effects of Ostad's energy: changes in DHEA, changes in EEG, changes in cardiac output and changes in the molecular structure of water. Obviously none of these particular measurements in itself proves or disproves "healing." Healing can be measured only in a patient's response symptomatically and/or with measurable changes in disease status. Nevertheless, these different tests provide strong evidence of Ostad Hadi Parvarandeh's unique ability to reinforce the many medical histories that document his effectiveness in treating many different types of disease as well as patients' reports of feeling energized when consuming Ostad's water, raisins or sugar cubes.

As I indicated earlier, when we first met Ostad my intent was to see what effect he would have on DHEA (dehydroepiandrosterone), the most prevalent hormone in the body, which, as I've already mentioned, is reduced in every known illness. It has been my belief from my own observations that the decline in DHEA is related to cumulative stress and how well individuals handle this.

When Ostad laid hands on twelve individuals, three times per person over a period of three consecutive days, the DHEA went up modestly in only two persons. In two there was no change, and in the other eight there was a DHEA decrease of 50–75 percent. This was totally in conflict with my hypothesis. The answer seemed to come from the one man in whom there had been an elevated PSA, or prostate specific antigen. This fifty-eight-year-old man was diagnosed with cancer of the prostate just two weeks earlier and had had two elevated PSAs. Interestingly, this man's PSA dropped about 65 percent at the same time that his DHEA began a modest drop. (His DHEA came back up slowly over the next several months.) The question is, did Ostad alter the DHEA? I think we can state that his interventions *affected* DHEA in ten out of twelve people, or more than 80 percent of individuals. That is quite remarkable because DHEA does not change more than 15 percent under ordinary circumstances from day to day, season to season, or from hour to hour. The probability is that Ostad *mobilized* DHEA in some way and put it to work doing something useful. In the patient with prostate cancer, the useful event appeared to be affecting the negative antigenic aspect of his prostate cancer.

MORE EVIDENCE OF SACRED HEALING

Twenty-five years ago I started out to find twenty-five cases of sacred healing. Despite my intense effort, I was able to collect less than a dozen proven cases until meeting Ostad Hadi Parvarandeh. This one remarkable healer has now provided one hundred medical records of his miraculous healing. I have scientifically documented medical records of remarkable cures in more than one hundred patients with various illnesses ranging from brain tumors and cancer to diabetes.

In other parts of this book, I've chronicled various cases of sacred healing. Here are some others I can report as a result of my work with Ostad.

- A thirty-eight-year-old woman with breast cancer metastatic to bone was pronounced cured after treatment by Ostad.
- Medical records from a leading American neurosurgeon reveal that a forty-six-year-old man with a spinal cord tumor diagnosed by MRI (magnetic resonance imaging) was healed with disappearance of the tumor and perhaps slight residual scar two years after treatment by Ostad.
- A woman with a cystic lesion of the pineal had the cyst completely disappear after healing by Ostad.
- Additional medical records confirm that Ostad healed patients with osteogenic sarcoma, the most malignant form of cancer, not curable with any chemotherapy; neuroblastoma in a six-month-old child; adenocarcinoma of the stomach in a sixty-six-year-old man

(stomach cancer is rarely cured with surgery or chemotherapy); spinal cord tumor not curable medically; hepatitis within ten days, with liver enzymes returning to normal; a ruptured intervertebral disc for which only surgery had been recommended; 40 percent recovery of visual fields in a man who originally was approximately 90 percent blind from retinitis pigmentosa; severe glaucoma (cured from a long distance); Hepatitis B; and Gilles de la Tourette's syndrome.

From a medical point of view, each of these cases represents a "white crow"—something that's not supposed to happen.

Working with Ostad culminates my search for documentation and scientific work that began twenty years ago with Olga Worrall. The case studies show an extensive and compelling series of scientifically documented effects. Most impressive, however, are the reports of thousands of patients—some of which I've presented here—most of whom had been failed by conventional medicine and healed through the focus of divine energy by this one great healer. A few other physicians in this country have also been privy to his work, and we have letters and records from some of them.

Alice Bailey, the great Theosophical writer, in her book

Esoteric Healing stated that healers often die young of heart disease or cancer. In October 1997, Ostad Hadi Parvarandeh died at the age of seventy-one. Despite his beliefs and despite his statement that the energy of ill persons did not affect him, seventy-one is young! It was apparent from my brief work with him that Ostad gave unconditionally and took little time for himself. Olga Worrall died in her late seventies; Edgar Cayce in his sixties. We must find ways to protect and prolong the life of talented Sacred Healers.

The future of sacred healing is dependent at this stage on organized, accredited training of other sacred healers. Those plans are in the works now. Though research has started, much remains to be done. Studies need to be done on diabetes, heart disease and other forms of cancer. The work of the Barbara Brennan School of Healing and the American Association of Spiritual Healers will be paramount in this future. Flocks of white crows will undoubtedly become common!

Endnotes

Introduction

1. Gina Cerinara, *Many Mansions* (New York: Signet Books, 1991), p. 82.

2. Ibid.

Chapter 1

1. William Nolen, *A Doctor in Search of a Miracle* (New York: Ballantine Books, 1947).

2. Ibid.

Chapter 2

1. John Cerroll Cruze, *The Incorruptibles* (Rockford, Ill.: Tan Books and Publishers, 1947).

2. All quotes in this section from William James, *The Varieties of*

Religious Experience (New York: Modern Library, 1936), pp. 77–124.

3. *Random House College Dictionary* (New York: Random House, 1984).

Chapter 4

1. Larry Dossey, *Prayer Is Good Medicine* (San Francisco: HarperSanFrancisco, 1996).

2. Franz Ingelfinger, "Health: A Matter of Statistics of Feeling" *New England Journal of Medicine*, February 24, 1977, pp. 448–49.

3. Sir William Osler, *Aequanimitas* (Philadelphia: Blakeston Company, 1943).

Chapter 5

1. Edwina Cerutti, *Olga Worrall: Mystic with Healing Hands* (New York: Harper and Row, Publishers, 1975).

2. For those who wish to contact Miatek Wirkus, his address is: Wirkus Bioenergy Foundation, 9907 E. Fleming Avenue, Bethesda, MD 20814, tel: 301-652-1691.

3. Rod Campbell, *Healing from Love: Healing through Love, Kindness, and Respect for All Living Things* (Auckland, New Zealand: Awareness Book Co., Ltd., 1996).

4. The guidelines for distinguishing the qualifications of and criteria for a master sacred healer I attained by way of extensive conversations with Ostad Hadi Parvarandeh, Grand Master Healer, and his wife, Fari.

Chapter 6

1. Evelyn Underhill, *The Spiritual Life* (New York: Penguin Books, 1993).

Chapter 7

1. Herbert Benson, "Angina Pectoris and the Placebo Effect," *New England Journal of Medicine*, 1979.

2. Norman Cousins, "Anatomy of an Illness (As Perceived by the Patient)," *New England Journal of Medicine*, 295:1458–63.

3. Randolph C. Byrd, "Positive Effects of Intercessory Prayer in a Coronary Care Unit Population," *Southern Medical Journal*, 81:7, July 1988, pp. 826–29.

Chapter 9

1. Robert O. Becker and Gary Selden, *The Body Electric: Electromagnetism in the Foundation of Life* (New York: William Morrow and Co., 1985).

2. Ibid.

3. Wilhelm Reich, *The Bioelectric Investigation of Sexuality and Anxiety* (New York: Farrar, Straus, and Ciroux, 1982).

4. Ibid.

5. Shealy, C. Norman; Helms, Joseph; and McDaniels, Allen. (December 1990). "Treament of male infertility with acupuncture." *The Journal of Neurological and Orthopaedic Medicine and Surgery*, Vol. 11, Issue 4, pp. 285–86.

Bibliography

1. Nolen, William A. *A Doctor in Search of a Miracle.* Ballentine Books, New York, 1974.

2. James, William. *The Varieties of Religious Experience.* Modern Library, New York 1902 (first modern library edition 1936).

3. Ingelfinger, Franz. "Health: A Matter of Statistics or Feeling." *New England Journal of Medicine,* pp. 448–49, February 24, 1977.

4. Cerutti, Edwina. *Olga Worrall: Mystic With the Healing Hands.* Harper and Rowe Publishers, New York, 1975.

5. Osler, Sir William. *Aequanimitas.* Blakeston Company, Philadelphia, 1943.

6. Dossey, Larry. *Prayer Is Good Medicine.* Harper, San Francisco, 1996.

7. Benson, Herbert. "Angina Pectoris and the Placebo Effect," *New England Journal of Medicine*, 1979.

8. Pelletier, Kenneth R. *Mind As Healer, Mind As Slayer.* Delacorte Press, New York, 1977.

9. Green, Elmer & Alyce. *Beyond Biofeedback.* Knoll Publishing, 1977.

10. Shealy, C. Norman. *90 Days to Self-Health.* Bantam Books, New York, 1977.

11. Justice, Blair. *Who Gets Sick.* St. Martin's Press, New York, 1988.

12. Underhill, Evelyn. *The Spiritual Life.* Penguin Books, New York, 1993.

13. *The New Lexicon Webster's Dictionary.* Lexicon Publications, Inc., New York, NY, 1987.

14. Cousins, Norman. "Anatomy of an Illness (As Perceived by the Patient). *New England Journal of Medicine* 295:1458–63, 1976.

15. Cousins, Norman. *Anatomy of an Illness As Perceived by the Patient.* W. W. Norton & Company, New York, 1979.

16. Davies, Robertson. *The Cunning Man.* Viking-Penguin, New York, 1996.

17. Becker, Robert O., and Selden Gary. *The Body Electric: Electromagnetism in the Foundation of Life.* William Morrow and Company, New York, NY, 1985.

18. Becker, Robert O., and Marino, Andrew A. *Electromagnetism and Life*. State University of New York Press, Albany, NY, 1982.

19. Reich, Wilhelm. *The Bioelectric Investigation of Sexuality and Anxiety*. Farrar, Straus, and Giroux, New York, NY, 1982.

20. Hammond, Sally. *We Are All Healers*. Ballentine Books, New York, 1974.

21. Campbell, Rod. *Healing From Love: Healing Through Love, Kindness, and Respect for All Living Things*, Awareness Book Co., Ltd., PO Box 9224, Newmark, Auckland, New Zealand, 1996.

22. Livingston-Wheeler, Virginia, and Addeo, Edmond G. *The Conquest of Cancer: Vaccines and Diet*. Waterside Productions, Inc., San Diego, CA, 1984.

23. Enby, Erik; Gosch, Peter; and Sheehan, Michael. *Hidden Killers: The Revolutionary Medical Discoveries of Professor Gunther Enderlein*. Semmelweis-Institute: Hoya, West Germany, 1990. (Available from Occidental Institute Research Foundation, Box 5507, Bellingham, WA 98227-5507.

24. Bird, Christopher. *The Galileo of the Microscope: The Life and Trial of Gaston Naessens*. Presses de L'Universite de La Bersonne, Inc., Saint Lambert, Quebec, Canada, 1990.

Books on a Positive Approach to Life

Shealy, C. Norman. *The Self-Healing Workbook*. Element Books, Boston, 1996.

Shealy, C. Norman and Myss, Caroline M. *The Creation of Health*. Stillpoint Publishing, Walpole, NH, 1993.